D1552474

Springer Series on
LIFE STYLES AND ISSUES IN AGING

Series Editor: Bernard D. Starr, PhD
Marymount Manhattan College
New York, NY

Advisory Board: Robert C. Athley, PhD; Marjorie Cantor, PhD (Hon); Harvey L. Sterns, PhD

1993 **RETIREMENT COUNSELING**
A Handbook for Gerontology Practitioners
Virginia E. Richardson, PhD

1994 **AGING AND QUALITY OF LIFE**
Ronald P. Abeles, PhD, Helen C. Gift, PhD, and Marcia G. Ory, PhD, MPH

1995 **IMPACT OF INCREASED LIFE EXPECTANCY**
Beyond the Gray Horizon
Mildred M. Seltzer, PhD

1995 **GEROCOUNSELING**
Counseling Elders and Their Families
Virginia S. Burlingame, MSW, PhD

1996 **LIFE BEYOND 85 YEARS**
The Aura of Survivorship
Colleen L. Johnson, PhD, and Barbara M. Barer, MSW

1999 **ETHNOGEROCOUNSELING**
Counseling Ethnic Elders and Their Families
Virginia S. Burlingame, MSW, PhD

1999 **WORKING WITH TOXIC OLDER ADULTS**
A Guide to Coping with Difficult Elders
Gloria M. Davenport, PhD

1999 **PRESERVATION OF THE SELF IN THE OLDEST YEARS**
With Implications for Practice
Sheldon S. Tobin, PhD

2000 **TO GRANDMOTHER'S HOUSE WE GO AND STAY**
Perspectives on Custodial Grandparents
Edited by Carole B. Cox, PhD

2000 **EMPOWERING GRANDPARENTS RAISING GRANDCHILDREN**
A Training Manual for Group Leaders
Carole B. Cox, PhD

2000 **ELDERS, CRIME, AND THE CRIMINAL JUSTICE SYSTEM**
Myth, Perceptions, and Reality in the 21st Century
Edited by Max B. Rothman, JD, LLM, Burton D. Dunlop, PhD, and Pamela Entzel, JD

2003 **SUCCESSFUL AGING AND ADAPTATION WITH CHRONIC DISEASES**
Edited by Leonard W. Poon, PhD, Dr Phil, hc, Sara Hall Gueldner, DSN, FAAN, and Betsy M. Sprouse, PhD

Leonard W. Poon, PhD, Dr Phil, hc, is Professor of Psychology; Chair, Faculty of Gerontology, and Director, Gerontology Center at the University of Georgia. He is a fellow of APA, APS, GSA, and AGHE. Among his ten edited books in gerontology are *Aging in the 1980s: Psychological Issues, Handbook for Clinical Assessment of Older Adults,* and *Everyday Cognition in Adulthood and Later Life.* He is one of the editors of the *Encyclopedia of Aging* published in 1986, 1995, and 2001 by Springer Publishing. His work in aging over the last 30 years included normal and pathological memory, clinical memory assessment, longevity and survival of the oldest-old and successful aging in the face of multiple chronic diseases.

Sarah Hall Gueldner, DSN, FAAN, is Professor of Nursing and Director, School of Nursing at The Pennsylvania State University. A fellow of Sigma Theta Tau and the American Academy of Nursing and a member of the Pennsylvania Geriatric Education Center, she is experienced in the training of nurses and other health care professionals in geriatrics. Dr. Gueldner has edited a number of books on health care and aging, with a recent publication on osteoporosis published by Springer Publishing and *Gerontological Nursing Issues for the 21ˢᵗ Centenary.*

Betsy M. Sprouse, PhD, is a Program Manager at the AARP Andrus Foundation in Washington, DC, where she directs the funding programs for gerontological research and the education and training of students in aging. She received her doctorate from the University of Wisconsin–Madison in adult education and gerontology, and has worked in the field of aging for almost 30 years. She is active in the Gerontological Society of America and is a Fellow of the Association for Gerontology in Higher Education, and makes frequent presentations at the annual meetings of these organizations on gerontological training issues and on funding for gerontological research. She is the author or editor of two dozen publications, including *Gerontology in Higher Education: Developing Institutional and Community Strength,* and *Impact of Foundation Funding in Aging on Professional and Institutional Development.*

Successful Aging
and **Adaptation** with
Chronic Diseases

Leonard W. Poon, PhD, D Phil hc
Sarah Hall Gueldner, DSN, FAAN
Betsy M. Sprouse, Phd
Editors

 Springer Publishing Company

Springer Publishing Company, Inc.
536 Broadway
New York, NY 10012-3955

Acquisitions Editor: Ursula Springer
Production Editor: Pamela Lankas
Cover design by Joanne Honigman

03 04 05 06 07 / 5 4 3 2 1

Library of Congress Cataloging-in-Publication Data

Successful aging and adptation with chronic diseases / Leonard W. Poon, Sara Hall Gueldner, Besty M. Sprouse, editors.
    p. cm.
    Includes bibliographical references and index.
    ISBN 0-8261-1975-1
    1. Aged—Health and hygiene. 2. Aged—Medical care. 3. Chronic diseases. I. Poon, Leonard W., 1942– II. Gueldner, Sarah Hall. III. Sprouse, Betsy M. IV. Springer series on life styles and issues in aging.

RA564.8.S825 2003
613'.0438—dc21

                                                                2003042487

Printed in the United States of America by Maple-Vail Book Manufacturing Group.

Contents

Foreword   *vii*

Preface   *ix*

Contributors   *xi*

1   Self-Rated Successful Aging: Correlates and Predictors   1
     William J. Strawbridge and Margaret I. Wallhagen

2   Successful Aging and Reciprocity Among Older Adults   25
     in Assisted Living Settings
     William Rakowski, Melissa A. Clark, Susan C. Miller, and
     Katherine M. Berg

3   Successful Aging: Intended and Unintended Consequences   55
     of a Concept
     Robert L. Kahn

4   Health Expectancy: An Indicator of Successful Aging and   70
     a Measure of the Impact of Chronic Disease and Disability
     Eileen M. Crimmins, Jung Ki Kim, and Aaron Hagedorn

5   Risk and Protective Factors for Physical Functioning   83
     in Older Adults With and Without Chronic Conditions:
     MacArthur Studies of Successful Aging
     Teresa Seeman and Xinguang Chen

6   Health Expectancy, Risk Factors, and Physical Functioning   104
     Janice Penrod and Peter Martin

7   Coping with Comorbidity   116
     Leonard W. Poon, Lynn Basford, Clare Dowzer, and
     Andrew Booth

8 Coping with Specific Chronic Health Conditions   151
   *Lynn Basford, Leonard W. Poon, Clare Dowzer, and
   Andrew Booth*

9 Managing Multiple Chronic Health Conditions in   181
   Everyday Life
   Janice Penrod, Sarah Hall Gueldner, and Leonard W. Poon

10 Coping with Multiple Chronic Health Conditions   209
    Peter Martin

11 Metanarratives Surrounding Successful Aging: 220
    The Medium Is the Message
    Ann L. Whall and Frank D. Hicks

References   *228*

Index   *255*

Foreword

An inevitable reality about the aging processes is that many older adults will likely confront an increased risk of developing one or more chronic diseases. The purpose of this book is to review, consolidate, and extend our current knowledge on successful aging, particularly on older persons' perceptions of, and adaptations to, chronic illnesses.

The chapters are designed to complement one another while addressing issues that are both theoretically and practically challenging. This book addresses several basic questions. How do older adults confront and cope with multiple health problems in their everyday lives? What are their perceptions of the impact of diseases on their successful aging? What is successful aging within this context? How do we measure the impact of chronic diseases? What are the risk and protective factors in relation to successful health maintenance among community-dwelling older adults? How do extant models and theories of coping deal with these practical issues?

The book contains three major sections, which respond to the preceding questions. An integration chapter follows each section. In the first section, chapters 1 and 2 address what we can learn about successful aging from those who are experiencing it, taking into account chronic health conditions. Chapter 1 used data from the Alameda County Study, a continuing longitudinal study begun in 1965, and chapter 2 presents data obtained from assisted-living residents and staff to explore reciprocity among older adults. Chapter 3 integrates the findings with extant theories of successful aging.

In the second section, chapters 4 examines how the impact of chronic diseases and disability can be measured by using national data sets, and chapter 5 examines risk and protective factors pertaining to physical functioning that were obtained through the MacArthur Studies of

Successful Aging. Chapter 6 discusses and integrates the findings on health expectancy, risk factors, and physical functioning.

In the third section, chapters 7 through 9 review the literature on coping with comorbidity and specific major health conditions, as well as data and models on how older adults cope with comorbidity in their everyday lives. Chapter 10 identifies, integrates, and extends pertinent concepts in these three chapters. Finally, chapter 11 concludes the book by reviewing and commenting on our knowledge and theories of successful aging from the perspectives of several philosophies of scientific inquiry.

A compendium to this book has also been published to summarize the findings in lay terms so that the research can be applied to everyday situations. This compendium has been produced by the AARP Andrus Foundation, which supported the five studies reported in this book. Both publications are planned for release at the same time.

The authors and editors are indebted to the AARP Andrus Foundation for funding the research described in this book and for their invitational conference February 15–17, 2002, which enabled us to present and discuss the findings of our studies.

The editors also appreciate the input of Hazel Hunley for her copyediting contributions, as well as the assistance of staff and students at the University of Georgia Gerontology Center and at the Pennsylvania State University School of Nursing, and especially the AARP Andrus Foundation for helping to make this book a reality.

Leonard W. Poon
Sarah Hall Gueldner
Betsy M. Sprouse

Preface

In 1998, the AARP Andrus Foundation, a grantmaking organization in Washington, DC, redesigned its funding priorities to focus on two issues of critical importance to the older population: Living with chronic health conditions, and aging and living environments. The AARP Andrus Foundation had supported gerontological research for 30 years, but since this shift in focus it began concentrating on finding solutions to the challenges that older adults may face as they age and try to remain independent.

One of the issues that has received attention because of this new funding priority is *successful aging*. This is a term that is not always easy to define, but the Foundation's concern has been the role of chronic health conditions and living environments in successful aging. For most older adults, the ideal of successful aging is to be healthy and to live independently in their own homes. But if they are unable to do so, can they still feel they are aging successfully?

The AARP Andrus Foundation began funding research to address this question in 1999 and provided support for the five research studies described in this book. Each takes a different slant on the issue of successful aging, but the common theme is the role of chronic health conditions in relation to successful aging. The five studies might well have been conducted and reported separately had it not been for a proposal in 2001 from the University of Georgia Gerontology Center to integrate the results of these studies into this book.

This is the first effort by the AARP Foundation to synthesize and disseminate the results of several grants on related topics. We are very pleased with the outcome, and hope that you find it valuable as well. From this type of research synthesis, we can gain a greater understanding of how older adults use certain coping mechanisms to live with different chronic health conditions in different environments, and how their definitions of successful aging may or may not be hindered by their physical health status.

We also invite you to visit our Web site at www.aarp.org/foundation for information on the AARP Foundation's grant programs and to see the results of other studies on issues of importance to the lives of older adults.

Betsy M. Sprouse, PhD
AARP Foundation

Contributors

Lynn Basford MA, BA(hons), RGN, NDN, PWT, RNT, Cert. Ed.
Professor and Head of Nursing
School of Health and
   Community Studies
University of Derby, Mickleover
   Campus
Derby, United Kingdom

Katherine M. Berg, PhD, PT
Associate Professor and Associate
   Director
School of Physical and
   Occupational Therapy
McGill University
Montreal, Quebec, Canada

Andrew Booth, BA, MSc., Dip. Lib., MCILIP
Senior Lecturer in Evidence
   Based Healthcare Information
School of Health and Related
   Research (ScHARR)
University of Sheffield
Sheffield, United Kingdom

Xinguang Chen, MD, PhD
Assistant Professor of Research
Department of Preventive
   Medicine
University of Southern
   California Keck School of
   Medicine
Los Angeles, California

Melissa A. Clark, PhD, MPH
Assistant Professor of
   Community Health
Department of Community
   Health and
Center for Gerontology and
   Health Care Research
Brown University
Providence, Rhode Island

Eileen M. Crimmins, PhD
Edna M. Jones Professor of
   Gerontology
Andrus Gerontology Center
University of Southern
   California
Los Angeles, California

Clare Dowzer, PhD
Research Associate
University of Sheffield
Sheffield, United Kingdom

Aaron Hagedorn, MA, MS
Project Manager, USC/UCLA
 Center on Biodemography
 and Population Health
Andrus Gerontology Center
University of Southern
 California
Los Angeles, California

Frank D. Hicks, PhD, RN
Assistant Professor
Niehoff School of Nursing
Loyola University Chicago
Chicago, Illinois
Postdoctoral Fellow
Center for Enhancement and
 Restoration of Cognitive
 Function
School of Nursing
University of Michigan
Ann Arbor, Michigan

Robert L. Kahn, PhD
Professor Emeritus, Department
 of Psychology and School of
 Public Health
Research Scientist Emeritus
 Institute for Social Research
University of Michigan
Ann Arbor, Michigan

Jung Ki Kim, PhD
Research Assistant Professor of
 Gerontology
Andrus Gerontology Center
University of Southern California
Los Angeles, California

Peter Martin, PhD
Director
Gerontology Program
Iowa State University
Ames, Iowa

Susan C. Miller, PhD, MBA
Assistant Professor of
 Community Health
Department of Community
 Health and
Center for Gerontology and
 Health Care Research
Brown University
Providence, Rhode Island

Janice Penrod, PhD, RN
Assistant Professor
School of Nursing
Pennsylvania State University
University Park, Pennsylvania

William Rakowski, PhD
Professor of Medical Science
Department of Community
 Health and
Center for Gerontology and
 Health Care Research
Brown University
Providence, Rhode Island

Teresa Seeman, PhD
Professor of Medicine and
 Epidemiology
Division of Geriatrics
University of California Los
 Angeles School of Medicine
Los Angeles, California

William J. Strawbridge, PhD, MPH
Senior Research Scientist
Human Population Laboratory
Public Health Institute
Berkeley, California

Margaret I. Wallhagen, PhD, RN, CS
Associate Professor
Department of Physiological Nursing
School of Nursing
University of California
San Francisco, California

Ann L. Whall, PhD, RN, FAAN
Fulbright Distinguished Scholar
Professor School of Nursing and Associate Director of the Michigan Geriatrics Center
University of Michigan
Ann Arbor, Michigan

Chapter 1

Self-Rated Successful Aging: Correlates and Predictors

William J. Strawbridge and Margaret I. Wallhagen

The concept of successful aging was proposed by John Rowe and Robert Kahn (1987) to separate the effects of disease from the aging process itself. As initially proposed, people who aged successfully would show little or no age-related decline in physiologic function, while people aging in the usual sense would show disease-associated decrements that are often interpreted as the effects of age. In a subsequent publication, Rowe and Kahn (1998) broadened their definition to include three criteria: avoiding disease and disability, maintaining physical and mental functioning, and being actively engaged with life. The third category includes being connected to other people and engaging in "productive" activities.

Although the concept of successful aging is attractive and directly challenges the view that aging inevitably involves unrelenting declines, it has proven difficult to operationalize. The criterion of little or no age-related decrements in physiologic function for those aging successfully can lead to focusing on a small, elite segment of the population and thus reduce interest in secondary and tertiary prevention for the majority of older persons already experiencing chronic conditions and symptoms. As noted by Edward Masoro (2001), the concept of successful aging could even undermine efforts to support care for chronic conditions associated with the increasing number of older persons because of the mistaken belief that lifestyle changes will "en-

1

able those reaching advanced ages to avoid the disabilities that are so costly in terms of societal resources" (p. 418).

The media's depiction of "super elders" such as senior marathon runners, who perform athletic feats that even most young persons cannot, may exacerbate the problem for those who are suffering ill effects of aging. Focusing on superior physical performance marginalizes many older persons by recognizing as successful only those who exhibit the same physical capabilities as athletic, younger persons. Also, it is not necessarily the case that risk factor patterns observed in such an elite group will lead to useful interventions for the rest of the older population. Finally, the word *successful* is problematic because it implies a contest in which there are winners and losers; however, most gerontologists are not ready to call someone a loser merely because he or she is diagnosed with arthritis. And who is comfortable being called unsuccessful? Concern about the use of the word has led some researchers to substitute different terms, such as *healthy aging, aging well,* or *productive aging* (Baltes, 1994; Butler & Gleason, 1985; LaCroix, Newton, Leveille, & Wallace, 1997), though each of these designations presents similar conceptual difficulties.

Nevertheless, there is increasing interest in health promotion and disease prevention in older persons, and interest in successful aging shifts the focus to older persons who are doing well as opposed to the usual focus on the four Ds (disease, disability, dementia, and death). This concept thus encourages an examination of the factors that enable positive health or aging.

Most researchers studying successful aging have followed Rowe and Kahn's model by selecting older persons who have minimal disability or high levels of physical functioning. Guralnik and Kaplan (1989) considered subjects to be aging successfully who scored in the top 20% on a combined physical function and exercise scale. The MacArthur Studies of Successful Aging included 70– to 79–year-olds who answered at least six of nine mental status questions correctly, remembered at least three of six elements of a short story, reported no disabilities on any of seven activities of daily living (ADLs), had no more than one disability on eight mobility and physical performance items, were able to hold a semi-tandem balance for at least 10 seconds, and were able to stand from a seated position five times within 20 seconds (Berkman, et al., 1993). To meet Roos and Havens' (1991) criteria for successful aging, subjects had to survive for 12 years following the baseline interview, live in community, receive fewer than 60 days of home care services in the last year, report fair or better perceived health, be able to walk outdoors, score well on a mental status test, have a state of mind no worse than "a bit weak," not need help for five activities of daily living or to go outdoors, and not use a wheelchair. Some of these standards seem arbitrary. The 12–year survival requirement in the Roos and Havens criteria also makes it likely that they are constructing a model of longevity rather than a paradigm of successful aging.

Several analyses of successful aging have followed Schmidt's (1994) more modest definition of it as "minimal interruption of usual function, although minimal signs and symptoms of chronic disease may be present" (p. 4). One study based on data from the Alameda County Study (Berkman & Breslow, 1983) used Schmidt's approach to define people who are aging successfully as needing no assistance or not having difficulty on any of 13 activity/mobility measures, yet who may have a little difficulty on five other measures: lifting or carrying weights over 10 pounds; stooping, crouching or kneeling; pushing or pulling a large object; lifting arms above the shoulders, and writing or handling small objects (Strawbridge, Cohen, Shema, & Kaplan, 1996). By this standard, 58% of subjects 65 years old or older were classified as aging successfully. In a similar vein, Manton and Stallard (1991) used 27 measures, including activities of daily living, instrumental activities of daily living, physical performance, and mobility measures to define six disability profiles; the highest profile (functionally unimpaired) constituted 32% of their sample.

Another approach is based on the model proposed by Baltes and Baltes, which describes successful aging as doing the best with what one has (Baltes & Carstensen, 1996). Other more broadly based approaches follow either the definition of Schmidt and allow for the presence of chronic disease at least in a mild form; or Baltes and Baltes who allow for an even more serious form (Kaplan & Strawbridge, 1994). In these models, successful aging is a more attainable goal than in the more restrictive models that apply to the small proportions of older persons who enter old age unscathed. However, with the exception of Baltes and Baltes, all of these models focus on physical functioning. They also imply an all-or-nothing categorization, whereas there is considerable evidence that the physical functioning capabilities of older persons vary over relatively short periods of time; disability, for example, is by no means always permanent (Manton, 1988).

Studies that have examined predictors of successful aging have identified factors such as exercise, frequent contact with other persons, absence of chronic disease, not smoking, and not being depressed as important (Benfante, Reed, & Brody, 1985; Guralnik & Kaplan, 1989; Roos & Havens, 1991; Rowe & Kahn, 1998).

The major factor missing from all these divergent views of successful aging, however, is what older persons themselves have to say. Rarely are older persons asked directly to take part in defining successful aging based on their own experience. Their roles are usually passive and involve responding to what researchers themselves have defined as successful aging. Surely those involved in the process of aging themselves should have insights based upon their own experiences that could prove invaluable. The experience of researchers at the Human Population Laboratory suggests that when older persons are asked about what is important in old age, they rate physical functioning as no more important in their own lives than other major aspects of life, such as social relationships, community ties, mental health, and continued learning. If this is so, successful aging could occur in the presence of chronic illness and involve growth-enhancing experiences. Such a perspective may involve doing the best with what one has in ways that go well beyond simple physical functioning.

On the other hand, there is also evidence that disease and disability drive many other aspects of life for older persons, such as mental health, frequency of activities outside the home, and not feeling left out. It is thus possible that older persons who rate other aspects of life as equal to or more important than physical functioning and disability are those who have not experienced difficulties with chronic illness. Perhaps older persons who succeed at aging in spite of chronic disease are the exception.

Research Questions

To shed light on what successful aging really means to those experiencing it, our study directly asked 899 older persons to classify themselves as aging successfully or not. Because these people were already enrolled in the long-running, longitudinal Alameda County Study, a large amount of additional information was available for us to examine regarding health, quality of life, important activities, and prior predictors of successful aging. Specific research questions examined for our study were as follows.

1. What proportion of older persons describe themselves as aging successfully?

2. What characteristics do such persons have?

3. How strongly do chronic conditions affect self-rated successful aging?

4. How do quality of life outcomes and major activities differ between those who report aging successfully and those who do not?

5. What prior factors predict subsequent self-rated successful aging?

Methods

Our study was based on a survey of 899 men and women who had responded to a 1999 follow-up in the longitudinal Alameda County Study, which is described here briefly to provide background and to characterize the population of our study.

The Alameda County Study

The Alameda County Study is a longitudinal study of determinants of health and functioning, begun in 1965 (Berkman & Breslow, 1983). Alameda is a large urban California county and includes the cities of Berkeley and Oakland as well as a number of smaller towns. In 1965, the population of Alameda County was representative of the larger population of the United States in terms of gender, age, and minority representation. Subjects still enrolled in the study remain representative of the older, community-dwelling population of the United States on a wide range of variables, including age, proportion Black, and prevalence of chronic conditions. The Alameda Study is unique in its combination of a large population base with no upper restrictions on age at entry; subjects remaining enrolled regardless of where they move or changes in their health condition; multiple waves of data collection; a rich array of behavioral, social, psychological, and sociodemographic measures, and follow-up extending more than three decades.

After the initial 1965 baseline study of 6,928 adults, follow-up surveys involving full ranges of data were conducted in 1974, 1983, 1994, and 1999. A follow-up focusing on physical and mental functioning was completed in 1995. Response rates for survivors have been extremely high, ranging from 85% to 97%. The figure for the 1999 follow-up was nearly 96%. Nearly half of those enrolled still resided in Alameda County, and nearly 75% lived in one of the counties surrounding San Francisco Bay.

Data

Subjects aged 65 or older who had responded to the 1999 follow-up questionnaire in the Alameda County Study were sent an additional questionnaire of ours with specific questions about successful aging. A total of 899 men and women aged 65 to 99 responded for a response rate of 87%. All completed the questionnaire asking them to rate their own successful aging status, what types of activities they were involved in, how strongly they felt in control of what was happening to them, how they evaluated their own quality of life, and some general questions concerning what was good about getting older, what was difficult, and what changes they would make in their lives if they had them to live over. In addition, we selected 50 for in-depth interviews to better understand how they were deciding whether or not they were aging successfully and what advice they might have for those coming down the road behind them.

Because our analyses have not been completed on the in-depth interviews, the results presented in this chapter focus on the quantitative results from analysis of the data derived from the responses to the questionnaire.

Measures Used

Successful Aging

Subjects were asked how strongly they agreed or disagreed with the statement "I am aging successfully (or aging well)." Response categories were *agree strongly, agree somewhat, disagree somewhat,* or *disagree strongly.* Sensitivity analyses on a variety of outcome measures indicated that those agreeing somewhat were more similar to those who disagreed somewhat or strongly with the statement than to those who agreed strongly, so only those who agreed strongly were classified as aging successfully; all other responses were classified as not aging successfully.

Physical Health and Disability

Chronic conditions included a count of the presence in the last 12 months of arthritis, asthma, bronchitis, cancer, diabetes, emphysema, heart disease, osteoporosis, peripheral artery disease, and stroke. Symptoms included a count of the presence in the last 12 months of high blood pressure, constant coughing or frequent colds, trouble breathing or shortness of breath, pain in the heart or tightness or heaviness in the chest, stomach pains, foot problems, leg cramps, dizziness, headaches, or getting very tired in a short time. For self-rated health, the subjects were asked whether their health was excellent, good, fair, or poor. Being classified as mobility impaired included having a lot of difficulty or requiring help with either climbing one flight of stairs or walking one-quarter mile.

Mental Health

The measure of depression was a set of 12 items that operationalized the diagnostic criteria for a major depressive episode outlined in *Diagnostic and Statistical Manual of Mental Disorders,* (DSM-IV-R) (American Psychiatric Association, 1994). Subjects who experienced five or more symptoms of depression almost every day for the previous 2 weeks, including disturbed mood (feeling sad, blue, or depressed) or anhedonia (loss of interest or pleasure in most things) were classified as experiencing a major depressive episode.

Activities in Old Age

Subjects were asked about involvement with family, enjoying intimacy, improving in something, having good health, staying mentally alert, growing spiritually, being involved with friends, doing good things for others, learning something new, being athletic, being physically fit, and being involved with groups or organizations. All questions used an "I" format, such as "I am involved with family" or "I am learning something new." The response set included *agree strongly, agree somewhat, disagree somewhat,* and *disagree strongly.* Similar to successful aging, scoring was *agree strongly* versus the other responses.

Health Behaviors

Physical activity was measured with a scale based upon five questions: frequency of physical exercise, taking part in active sports, taking long walks, gardening, and swimming. The response set for each item was *never, sometimes,* or *often;* scoring was 0, 1, or 2, respectively. Scores on the scale ranged from 0 to 10. A four-item version of this scale has been used in previous analyses demonstrating a protective effect for physical activity on all-cause and cardiovascular mortality (Kaplan, Strawbridge, Cohen, & Hungerford, 1996; Strawbridge, Cohen, Kurata, & Kaplan, 2000). For cigarette smoking, the subjects were classified as *never, former,* or *current* smokers. Following new guidelines from the National Heart, Lung, and Blood Institute (1998), obesity was based upon a body mass index (BMI) of 30 or higher. The number of servings of fruits and vegetables eaten each day was scored five or more versus five or fewer, based on a single question asking subjects to fill in the number.

Quality of Life

This was assessed with depression (already described above), six other dichotomous measures, and three scales assessing optimism, psychological well-being, and cynical distrust. Global quality of life was determined using a version of Cantril's Ladder in which subjects were asked to rate their present quality of life by selecting a number from a vertical axis numbered from 1 to 9 (Cantril, 1965). Number 9 was labeled *Best old age I could expect;* number 7, *Good old age;* number 5, *Average old age;* number 3, *Not so good old age,* and number 1, *Worst old age I could expect.* Scale distribution was decidedly not normal, with responses clustered toward the high end, so for the analyses here the scale was dichotomized at 8 or 9 (*best old age*) versus all lower responses. Other dichotomous measures and scoring were as follows: pleased how life turned out (*strongly agree* versus *somewhat agree or disagree*), much more energy than others (versus *a little more, a little less,* or *a lot less*), very happy (versus *pretty* or *not too*), enjoy free time a lot (versus *some* or *not very much*), and very much feel loved and cared about (versus *somewhat, little,* or *very little*).

Optimism was measured by the revised version of the Life Orientation Test (Scheier, Carver, & Bridges, 1994). The six items in the scale are equally divided between those worded in a positive direction (such as "I'm always optimistic about my future") and those worded in a negative or pessimistic direction (such as "I hardly ever expect things to go my way"). Scoring is with a 4-point Likert scale ranging from 0 (*strongly disagree*) to 3 (*strongly agree*). Negative items were reverse coded so that higher scores reflected higher optimism. Scores ranged from 0 to 18. Cronbach's alpha was 0.73, relatively close to the 0.78 reported by the scale's developers who used college students as subjects (Scheier et al., 1994).

Bradburn's Affect Balance Scale was used to assess psychological well-being (Bradburn, 1969) among the Alameda sample. Four items measure positive affect (such as "Pleased about having accomplished something"), and four measure negative affect (such as "So restless you couldn't sit long in a chair)." Subjects are asked how often they feel each way; scoring is with a 3-point Likert scale ranging from 0 (*never*) to 2 (*often*). Negative scores are subtracted from the positive scores. Standardized Cronbach's alpha is 0.74.

Cynical distrust was measured by seven of the eight items from the Cynical Distrust Scale (Greenglass & Julkunen, 1989), which was itself developed from the much longer Cook-Medley Hostility Scale (Cook &

Medley, 1954). Response options used the same 4-point Likert Scale described for optimism. The seven items comprising the scale were as follows:

- It is safer to trust nobody.
- Most people make friends because friends are likely to be useful to them.
- I think most people would lie in order to get ahead.
- Most people inwardly dislike putting themselves out to help other people.
- No one cares much what happens to me.
- Most people are honest chiefly because of a fear of being caught.
- Most people will use somewhat unfair means to gain profit or an advantage rather than lose it.

The scale has a theoretical range of 0 to 21 with scores here ranging from 0 to 19; higher scores indicate greater cynical distrust. Cronbach's alpha was 0.81, identical to that reported by Cook and Medley for the eight-item version (Greenglass & Julkunen, 1989). This scale has been shown in another study to predict increased risk of both mortality and acute myocardial infarction among older males (Everson et al., 1997).

Social Relationships

Community involvement was measured by frequency of going out to volunteer (*often* versus *sometimes or never*). Relationship satisfaction was measured by asking how satisfied subjects were with their friendships and relationships with others; responses were coded *very* versus *somewhat* or *not at all*. Marital satisfaction was measured by asking married subjects how happy their marriage was; responses were coded *very happy* versus all other responses. Subjects with living children were asked whether any of their children were having problems with finances, employment, health, close relationships with others, or emotional problems. Those answering positively to any of the five problems were scored as having children who were having problems.

Religiosity and Spirituality

Attendance at religious services was scored as *weekly* versus *less* or *not at all*. Two items assessed spirituality. One asked how often subjects felt connected to others who may not share their faith. Coding was *very often* versus *often, sometimes,* or *never.* The other item asked how important spiritual values were "for what you do every day." Coding was *very important* versus *fairly important, a little important,* or *not at all important.*

Neighborhood and Financial Problems

Neighborhood problems were scored as a scale consisting of the number of neighborhood conditions reported by subjects as *somewhat* or *very serious problems*; conditions included crime, traffic, noise, trash and litter, night lighting, and availability of public transportation. Range of the scale was 0 to 6. Financial problems included any one of the following: not having enough money in the past 12 months to buy clothing, fill a prescription, see a doctor, pay rent or mortgage, or (in the last 30 days) buy food.

Hearing Impairment

Three questions asked how much difficulty subjects had, even with a hearing aid, hearing and understanding words in a normal conversation, hearing well enough to carry on a conversation in a noisy room, and hearing words clearly over the telephone. Response sets for each question were *a great deal* (3), *some* (2), *a little* (1), or *none* (0). Scores were summed with a resulting range of 0 to 9. This scale has been used in several research studies to analyze the impact of hearing impairment on subsequent health and functioning (Strawbridge, Wallhagen, Shema, & Kaplan, 2000; Wallhagen, Strawbridge, & Kaplan, 2001).

Vision Impairment

Three questions asked how much difficulty subjects had, even with glasses, seeing well enough to read street signs at night, recognize a friend across the street, or read a newspaper. Response sets and scoring were the same as for the hearing impairment scale just described. This scale has been used in a comparative analysis to assess the comparative impacts of hearing and vision impairment on a wide variety of functional outcomes (Wallhagen, Strawbridge, Shema, Kurata, & Kaplan, 2001).

Other Variables

Demographic variables included age in whole years, sex, ethnicity (White, Black, Asian, American Indian, or Hispanic), education (less than 12 years of education, 12 years, some college, or college graduate), and marital status (married, widowed, divorced/separated, or never married).

Risk factors from 1994 that were used for predicting successful aging in 1999 included a subset of the variables described above. All were measured the same way as their 1999 counterparts with the exception of cigarette smoking. Because the purpose in examining earlier risk factors was to focus on the health behaviors that potentially could be changed, 1994 cigarette smoking was measured simply as nonsmokers versus current smokers.

Analytic Strategies

To examine the characteristics of the people who were aging successfully, simple descriptive analyses were used according to demographic characteristics, self-rated health, number of chronic conditions, and number of symptoms.

Then the 11 activities and conditions were examined for those who are aging successfully and were compared with those who were not. Because there were some large gender differences on these activities and conditions, comparisons were also made between successfully aging men and women. Successful aging and gender differences were tested for statistical significance, using logistic models that adjusted for age. For these tests, the activity or condition was entered as the dependent variable with either age and successful aging or age and gender entered as independent variables.

Next the analyses focused on the extent to which those aging successfully also reported higher quality of life. For the seven dichotomous variables, each quality of life measure was used in statistical models as the dependent variable with age, sex, and successful aging entered as independent variables. For the three continuous variables, each was entered as the dependent variable in separate multiple regression models with age, sex, and successful aging entered as independent variables.

Attributes of successful aging were analyzed by including successful aging as the dependent variable in logistic models with each of the health behaviors, social relationship, religiosity, spirituality, neighborhood, financial problems, and sensory impairment variables entered as independent variables. Two sequential models were used for each attribute. The first was adjusted for only age and gender, while the second was adjusted for age, gender, number of chronic conditions, and number of symptoms.

Finally, a series of analyses examined the likelihood of successful aging in 1999 based upon the number of positive factors in 1994. To determine the specific predictors to be used, the 1994 counterpart for each of the 1999 attributes that were significantly related to successful aging was examined. The six strongest predictors were these: having little or no hearing impairment, not smoking cigarettes, not being obese, being physically active, volunteering, and being satisfied with social relationships. These predictors were combined into a scale consisting of the number of positive factors reported; range was 0 to 6. Because of the strong impact of chronic conditions, the likelihood of successful aging based upon the number of positive 1994 factors was calculated for subjects reporting 0, 1, or 2 chronic conditions in 1994. For all of these analyses, logistic regression models were used, with successful aging in 1999 entered as the dependent variable, and age, sex, number of 1994 chronic conditions, and the number of positive 1994 factors entered as independent variables. To present these last results in more easily understood terms than odds ratios, the specific likelihood of aging successfully (expressed as a percentage) was calculated for 0 to 6 positive factors with 0, 1, or 2 chronic conditions. Age was entered as 75 years (the mean age of subjects in 1999), and separate results were calculated for men and for women.

All calculations were performed using SAS, Version 6.12 (SAS Institute, Cary, North Carolina).

Results

The results of the quantitative analyses are described below, along with five tables on the statistical results.

Self-Ratings on Aging Successfully

As Table 1.1 indicates, when the 899 subjects were asked to rate their own successful aging, they split down the middle with 49.8% strongly

Table 1.1 Characteristics of Participants and Percentage Aging Successfully

Characteristic	Number	Self-rated successful aging
All subjects	899	49.8
Gender		
Female	501	52.3
Male	398	46.7
Age		
65–69	236	56.4
70–79	473	49.7
80–89	171	42.7
90–99	19	36.8
Ethnicity		
White	780	50.4
Black	49	44.9
Asian	40	45.0
Hispanic	18	61.1
American Indian	12	33.3
Number of chronic conditions		
0	321	67.3
1	300	47.3
2	154	36.4
3 or more	124	27.4
Mobility impaired		
Yes	106	17.0
No	793	54.2
Education		
Less than 12 yrs 129	45.0	
High school grad 279	53.8	
Some college	229	45.9
College graduate	262	51.5
Marital status		
Married	588	51.7
Widowed	207	48.3
Divorced/separated	86	43.0
Never married	18	38.9

(cont.)

Table 1.1 *(Continued)*

Characteristic	Number	Self-rated successful aging
Self-rated health		
Excellent	204	79.9
Good	524	49.2
Fair	144	16.7
Poor	27	11.1
Number of symptoms		
0	278	62.6
1	262	57.2
2	157	45.2
3	97	30.9
4	52	25.0
5 or more	53	18.9

agreeing they were aging successfully and 50.2% not agreeing. Women (52.3%) were somewhat more likely than men (46.7%) to rate themselves as aging successfully, as were those who were married (51.7%) compared with those who were either widowed, never married, or divorced/separated. For ethnicity, White subjects were a little higher than Black or Asian subjects. Hispanic subjects had the highest percentage for successful aging (61.1%), while American Indians had the lowest at 33.3%. Small numbers, however, make these last two percentages unreliable. Education had a positive effect through high school graduation but no increase beyond that.

There were relatively large differences by age group. The percentage rating themselves as aging successfully went down with increasing age but was still 36.8% for those in their 90s.

The number of chronic conditions did play a role. Two thirds of those with no chronic conditions rated themselves as aging successfully; for those with one, two, and three or more chronic conditions the proportion of those aging successfully dropped to 47.3%, 36.4%, and 27.4%, respectively. There were also large differences by number of symptoms.

Self-rated health differences were large, with results ranging from 79.9% aging successfully for those reporting their health as excellent to only 11.1% for those reporting their health as poor.

Finally, mobility impairment was a factor as well. Only 17.0% of those with mobility impairment still rated themselves as aging successfully.

Thus, chronic conditions, symptoms, and general fitness are important, but they are by no means the whole story. Particularly notable in the data just presented is that fully one third of those with no chronic conditions still rated themselves as *not* aging successfully while significant segments of those with one, two, and even three or more chronic conditions said that they were.

Activities in Old Age

Table 1.2 presents data on 11 activities and conditions for two groups of subjects. The successful aging comparisons involve all subjects, while the gender comparisons involve only those 448 subjects who rated themselves as aging successfully. Statistically significant higher proportions of those aging successfully strongly agreed that they were doing all of the activities. However, among those aging successfully, relatively

Table 1.2 Self-Rated Successful Aging and Gender Comparisons in Activities and Conditions in Old Age

| Activity or condition | All subjects (%) | | Only those aging successfully | |
	Yes	No	Men	Women
Growing spiritually	41.3	21.0	28.9	50.2
Athletic	21.8	5.0	27.2	17.9
Involved with friends	69.8	37.0	61.4	75.7
Involved with groups	48.6	21.0	40.4	54.5
Doing good things for others	67.5	33.8	62.0	71.4
Enjoying intimacy	55.8	30.7	64.4	48.9
Physically fit	57.0	10.7	57.3	56.8
Involved with family	79.1	64.3	80.0	78.5
Staying mentally alert	84.1	48.0	82.3	85.4
Improving in something	49.6	18.6	48.0	50.8
Learning something new	53.6	15.4	51.4	55.2

Note: All observed differences for successful aging are statistically significant at $p <$ 0.05, using a logistic model adjusting for age as are the first six activities or conditions for gender.

large gender differences were noted for six of the activities. Women scored higher on growing spiritually, being involved with friends, being involved with groups, and in doing good things for others. Men scored higher in describing themselves as athletic and enjoying intimacy. Because older men are more likely than older women to still be married, the gender difference in intimacy was further tested using an additional logistic model adjusting for age, gender, and marital status; results indicated that the observed gender difference was still statistically significant. Regardless of marital status, the men were more likely than the women to strongly agree they were enjoying intimacy.

No gender differences were noted for being physically fit, having good health, being involved with family, staying mentally alert, improving in something, or in learning something new.

These results indicate that those aging successfully are more involved in a wide variety of activities but that the worlds of successful aging for men and women do not entirely overlap. Older women aging successfully appear more involved in personal and community relationships outside of family and in growing spiritually.

Quality of Life Comparisons

Tables 1.3 and 1.4 present the results comparing quality of life among those aging successfully with those who are not. Outcomes for the

Table 1.3 Quality of Life Outcomes Comparing Those Aging Successfully with Those Not (Dichotomous Measures)

Outcome	Odds ratio	95% confidence interval
Best possible old age	8.73	6.40 to 11.9
Pleased how life turned out	3.01	2.27 to 3.99
Much more energy than others own age	6.74	4.63 to 9.82
Very happy	3.62	2.70 to 4.86
Enjoy free time a lot	4.55	3.30 to 6.28
Very much feel loved and cared about	2.19	1.60 to 2.99
Depressed	0.26	0.16 to 0.45

Note: All models are adjusted for age and gender. All outcomes are statistically significant at $p < 0.05$.

Table 1.4 Quality of Life Outcomes Comparing Those Aging Successfully with Those Not (Continuous Measures)

Outcome	Regression coefficient	95% confidence interval
Life Orientation Test	1.77	1.38 to 2.16
Bradburn Affect Balance	3.01	2.27 to 3.99
Cynical distrust	−1.21	−0.67 to −1.75

Note: All models are adjusted for age and gender. All outcomes are statistically significant at $p < 0.05$.

dichotomous measures in Table 1.3 are expressed as odds ratios, which compare the likelihood of the indicated outcome (age and gender adjusted) for those aging successfully compared with those who are not. Thus the odds of being very happy were more than 3 times higher for those aging successfully. Large differences were also noted for the other outcomes. For depression, the odds ratio of 0.26 means that those aging successfully were much less likely to be depressed. None of the indicated 95% confidence intervals crosses 1.0, indicating that all of the results are statistically significant.

Results for the three continuous measures are shown in Table 1.4; the regression coefficients indicate the adjusted mean differences in scores for those aging successfully compared with those who were not. Those aging successfully scored an average 1.77 points higher on the Life Orientation Test, 1.74 points higher on the Affect Balance scale, and 1.21 points lower on the Cynical Distrust scale. These results indicate a more positive outlook on life, coupled with less distrust of the motives of others for those who rated themselves as aging successfully compared with those who did not.

Attributes of Successful Aging

Cross-sectional attributes in 1999 associated with successful aging are presented in Table 1.5. Two sets of models are shown; the first adjusts for only age and gender while the second adds the number of chronic conditions and number of symptoms.

Among the five health behaviors, only moderate alcohol consumption had no association with successful aging in the first set of models. When adjustments were added for number of chronic conditions and number of symptoms, the observed relationships weakened, with the

Table 1.5 Attributes of Self-Rated Successful Aging

Attribute	Model 1[a] OR (95% CI)	Model 2[b] OR (95% CI)
Health behaviors		
Never smoked cigarettes	1.40 (1.07–1.84)	1.13 (0.85–1.50)
Obese	0.63 (0.43–0.92)	0.87 (0.58–1.31)
Physical Activity Scale	1.36 (1.26–1.45)	1.27 (1.18–1.37)
Moderate alcohol consumption	1.11 (0.84–1.46)	1.02 (0.76–1.36)
5 or more daily servings of vegetables	1.44 (1.08–1.91)	1.30 (0.96–1.75)
Social relationships		
Often volunteer	2.12 (1.44–3.12)	1.92 (1.28–2.87)
Satisfied with relationships	2.42 (1.77–3.31)	2.17 (1.56–3.02)
Marriage very happy[c]	1.86 (1.33–2.61)	1.69 (1.19–2.39)
Children having problem[d]	0.72 (0.54–0.94)	0.93 (0.69–1.25)
Religiosity and spirituality		
Attend religious services weekly	1.06 (0.79–1.42)	1.04 (0.76–1.41)
Often feel connected to others who may not share my faith	1.70 (1.28–2.24)	1.72 (1.28–2.31)
Spiritual values very important for what I do every day	1.42 (1.08–1.87)	1.41 (1.06–1.88)
Neighborhood and financial problems		
Neighborhood problems scale	0.76 (0.64–0.89)	0.81 (0.68–0.97)
Any financial problems	0.50 (0.30–0.82)	0.64 (0.37–1.10)
Sensory impairment		
Hearing impairment scale	0.88 (0.83–0.93)	0.91 (0.86–0.97)
Vision impairment scale	0.88 (0.82–0.93)	0.92 (0.86–0.99)

[a]Adjusted for age and gender
[b]Adjusted for age, gender, number of chronic conditions, and number of symptoms
[c]For married subjects only
[d]For subjects with children only

exception of physical activity. Results were somewhat different for the four social relationship variables where only children having problems became not statistically significant when the additional adjustments were made.

Weekly attendance at religious services was not associated with successful aging, but the two variables representing spirituality were. Often feeling connected to others who may not share one's faith and feeling that spiritual values are very important for what one does every day revealed the same pattern: their statistically significant associations with successful aging when only age and gender adjustments were made were unaffected by adjustments for number of chronic conditions or number of symptoms.

The number of neighborhood problems as well as any financial problems reduced the likelihood of successful aging in the first set of models, but only the former remained associated with successful aging in the second set of adjustments.

Both hearing and visual impairment were associated with self-rated successful aging in both sets of models.

Five-Year Predictors of Successful Aging

As described in the Methods section, the attributes from Table 1.5 were examined using their 1994 values to develop a set of important positive factors to predict who would be more likely to be aging successfully 5 years later. The six attributes selected and the percentage of subjects doing each one in 1994 were the following: being physically active (31%), often volunteering (15%), being very satisfied with personal relationships (74%), having little or no hearing impairment (62%), not smoking (90%), and not being obese (86%). Some of these factors, of course, are easier to change than others, but all at least have the potential for improvement, and four of them were already being done by a majority of study participants.

Being physically active was represented by someone who often does at least one physical activity (e.g., going for long walks, exercising, playing a sport, or swimming) coupled with doing at least one additional activity sometimes or often. Little or no hearing impairment was represented by someone answering *never* to all three hearing impairment questions described in the Methods section, or *never* on two, and only *a little* on one other.

On how many of these six factors did the subjects score positively on in 1994? Most were positive on three or four, with about 20% actually doing five, and 13% only doing two. Only 4% were positive on all six, while only one subject was negative on all of them. Incidentally, he also rated himself as not aging successfully 5 years later.

We then used computer modeling to estimate the likelihood of successful aging in 1999 for study participants, based upon how many of the six positive factors they were doing 5 years earlier.

In order to express the results in percentages for likelihood of successful aging rather than odds ratios, it was necessary to specify

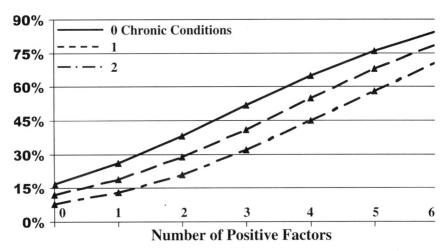

Figure 1.1 Likelihood of aging successfully by number of positive factors 5 years earlier: Woman at age 75.

age. For age we used 75 years, which represented the mean age of the subjects in the study.

Because chronic conditions are also important for successful aging, we calculated the likelihood of aging successfully for both 75–year-old men and women with 0, 1, or 2 chronic conditions. Results for women are shown in Figure 1.1.

The three lines indicate the likelihood of aging successfully for a 75–year old woman with various scores on the six positive factors from 5 years before and depending upon the number of chronic conditions reported.

Figure 1.2 provides the same information for a 75–year old man. Although the patterns are very similar for both men and women, the actual likelihood percentages for men are all just a little lower than for women.

Note (in Figures 1.1 and 1.2) that for both men and women all of the lines go up as the number of positive factors increases, but the likelihood of aging successfully is reduced as the number of chronic conditions increases. However, although the number of chronic conditions does make a difference, the increase in the likelihood of aging successfully for each increase in the number of positive factors is such that it balances the reduction associated with one additional chronic condition. Entering different ages into the computer models would have the following effects. Lower ages (such as age 65) would increase

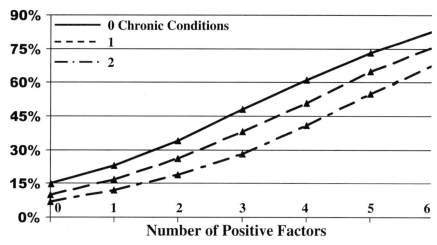

Figure 1.2 Likelihood of aging successfully by number of positive factors 5 years earlier: Man at age 75.

all of the likelihood figures, whereas higher ages (such as 80) would reduce them.

Discussion

Half of the older persons taking part in our study rated themselves as aging successfully, a much higher percentage than found in most other studies where researchers rather than subjects decide upon the criteria used to define successful aging. Nevertheless, the relatively strong associations between self-rated successful aging and chronic conditions, symptoms, self-rated health, physical fitness, and mobility impairment are consistent with the work of Rowe and Kahn and with the results of the other studies described in the introduction to this chapter, which stressed the importance of health and functioning for successful aging. It seems clear, therefore, that as chronic conditions and symptoms increase, the likelihood of successful aging decreases. Thus, indications are that avoiding disease and disability are important components of successful aging.

But what distinguishes our work from other studies is that, although optimal health and functioning do appear to be important for successful aging, they are by no means the entire story. About a third of our subjects with chronic conditions still rated themselves as aging successfully, while a third of those with no chronic conditions did not. Indeed, these subjects may hold the key to understanding what successful aging is all about because they are the inconsistent ones. Understanding why some older persons with multiple chronic conditions and symptoms still rate themselves as aging successfully, while some with no chronic conditions and no symptoms say they are not, could shed much light on what it means to age successfully.

The higher participation rates for those aging successfully on a wide variety of activities indicate a much more active involvement in life. The observed gender differences, however, indicate that older men and women emphasize somewhat different activities. The women are more involved in social relationships, community activities, and in spiritual growth, while the men are more likely to describe themselves as athletic and say that they are enjoying intimacy.

We also learned from our analyses that there are things we all can do now to increase our chances of aging successfully, that is, not smoke, be physically active, avoid obesity, protect hearing, maintain good personal relationships, and be active in community groups. Interestingly enough, each one of these activities had an impact on subsequent successful aging similar to having one less chronic condition. It may be that each of the factors acts both to reduce the likelihood of developing chronic conditions and to promote other positive health benefits. The association between these factors and successful aging should hold no surprises because all have been shown in other analyses to promote better health and (with the exception of avoiding hearing loss) longevity. The two social-relationship variables are also consistent with Rowe and Kahn's (1998) factor of active engagement with life.

Two of the factors we identified as predicting subsequent successful aging raise special concerns. The prevalence of obesity and hearing impairment have risen sharply in recent years (National Heart, Lung and Blood Institute, 1998; Wallhagen, Strawbridge, Cohen, & Kaplan, 1997), standing in marked contrast to the dramatic drop in cigarette smoking that has occurred. Indeed, as noted earlier, only 10% of older Alameda County Study subjects were still smoking cigarettes in 1994, while 14% were obese and 38% evidenced more than a little hearing impairment. Should these two latter factors continue to increase, the proportion of older persons aging successfully could decrease in future years.

Successful aging is more than an individual affair. Public policy has a role to play because all six positive factors as well as health can be enhanced by community action. Antismoking campaigns have already reduced the prevalence of smoking. In fact, 55% of the subjects in this study had smoked at one time in their lives compared with the 10% who were still doing so. Campaigns to increase physical activity may be reaching a larger number of people as well, but communities can facilitate the process by ensuring safe streets, appropriate facilities, and mechanisms for those who wish to exercise with others. The increasing prevalence of obesity and hearing impairment has already been discussed; the latter begs for further research in order to understand better why it is increasing and to prevent its occurrence and minimize its impact. Finally, the two social factors of volunteerism and individual relationships rest in part on communities that foster social connections rather than on the increasingly isolated lifestyles that seem typical of many modern Americans (Putnam, 2000).

Some cautions are in order. We do not know for sure the basis on which our subjects are rating themselves as aging successfully or not, nor do we know how stable such a statement is. Most of the results described here are also based upon cross-sectional data, which means it is impossible to say very much about causal order. We *do* know from our data that self-rated successful aging is consistent with a wide variety of positive quality-of-life measures, but we do not know which are causing what. Although we had earlier data for many variables, we had no earlier measure of successful aging. So it may be that a sense of successful aging causes better mental health and well-being, or it may be the reverse, or it may be that both successful aging and a higher quality of life are caused by something else that we did not measure. We did ask 50 of our subjects to talk about successful aging in much more detail, so it is possible that we will learn enough from these interviews to speak with more confidence. However, it will take a longitudinal analysis to really understand the process of successful aging. With such a design, successful aging can be measured both at the start and at the end of the study. Alternatively, a more complex study may be needed where the processes of moving toward or away from successful aging could be better understood. In such an analysis, the concept of successful aging would be more flexible than has been the case in previous research or in our own analyses here. Such work will take time.

In the meantime, we think the work presented here demonstrates the value of involving older persons themselves in discussing and understanding successful aging. After all, they are there now and have much to tell those who will follow.

Acknowledgments

This study was funded by a grant from the AARP Andrus Foundation. Support was also received from the National Institute on Aging (Grant 1R37AG11375) and by the Prevention Health Services block grant from the Centers for Disease Control and Prevention. The authors would like to acknowledge the analysis assistance of Richard D. Cohen and Sarah J. Shema.

Chapter 2

Successful Aging and Reciprocity Among Older Adults in Assisted Living Settings

William Rakowski, Melissa A. Clark,
Susan C. Miller, and Katherine M. Berg

The initial onset and subsequent day-to-day experiences of living with chronic health problems affect older adults' participation in social networks, challenge them to reexamine their self-concept, and require them to reevaluate the progression of their own aging process. Over the past 30 years, studies have shown that these tasks and challenges are common for older adults living with a variety of illnesses (e.g., stroke, chronic obstructive pulmonary disease, rheumatoid arthritis), and include testing the limits of impairments; dealing with uncertainties about treatment options and progress; deciding how much information about their situation to tell family members and health professionals; maintaining a balance between accepting help and retaining independence and control; and trying to maintain a feeling of contributing to a household and social network (Moos, 1984; Rakowski, 1984; Strauss & Glasser, 1975).

Individuals dealing with these issues are in an ambiguous situation. Because of the progressive but gradual nature of most chronic conditions, they experience impairment to some functions but can still maintain health and good performance in other domains. The steady increase over the past decades in life expectancy after reaching age 65 has resulted in greater numbers of persons living under these circumstances. In addition, the diversification of options in long-term care has allowed more persons to remain in the community rather than move to institutional settings. In essence, these people who are often very elderly are the pioneers of their generation. Their ability to remain in community-based residential settings pushes the boundaries that have been used to describe healthy aging, aging well, and even successful aging. In the 1960s and 1970s, it was novel to study concepts of health promotion and prevention among persons over age 75. Such research and service programs are now common. The concept of successful aging is now undergoing a similar evolution.

Previous Research on Successful Aging

Discussions and research on the topic of successful aging have become more visible in the gerontological literature since the mid 1980s. The 1987 article by Rowe and Kahn that drew a distinction between "usual aging" and "successful aging" was a major stimulus and, perhaps, was the capstone of its period, representing several themes that had begun to emerge. For example, Butler and Gleason (1985) had edited a volume of papers under the rubric of "productive aging," and Fries (1983) had advanced the premise of the compression of morbidity. In the early 1980s, social and behavioral epidemiologic research had begun to identify lifestyle predictors of "healthy aging," drawing on existing samples such as the Alameda County Study (Berkman & Breslow, 1983). The Established Populations for Epidemiologic Studies of the Elderly (EPESE) were also being established for long-term investigation (Coroni-Huntley, Brock, Ostfeld, Taylor, & Wallace, 1986). The concept of disability-free life expectancy was entering the literature on functional status as a positive complement to the traditional focus on difficulty with the ADL, IADL and Nagi-type activities of daily living. Research on the psychological processes of aging included results of prospective investigations such as the Seattle Longitudinal Study of Aging, which demonstrated sustained performance of some cognitive skills and contributed to subsequent research on the "plasticity" of aging (Schaie & Willis, 1986). Even earlier, the debate on Disengagement Theory versus Activity Theory and the classic distinction between crystallized and fluid intelligence can be seen as the efforts of gerontology in the

1960s to understand the nature of later life and to optimize its potential.

A major empirical and philosophical challenge has been to establish definitions of success that allow a broad range of older persons to be included, rather than to establish definitions that exclude groups of the population on a virtually a priori basis because they do not meet the criteria posed for optimal aging. For example, to the extent that productive, vital, and healthy aging in the postretirement years are defined by television commercial images (e.g., the 80–year-old water-skier, the creative artist producing potential masterpieces, or the world traveler thanking an investment company for financial security), a substantial percentage of older persons are excluded a priori from qualifying for classification as a successful older adult.

In addition, in much of the research done to date, successful aging has often been defined by a person's meeting or exceeding a standard based on the performance of relatively healthy people (Rakowski, Pearlman, & Murphy, 1995). Even if not presented directly in terms of meeting or beating an existing record, the implication is that successful aging is gauged by a comparison to peers, and perhaps even on a competitive model. The risk of a comparative or a competitive model is that only a select percentage of older persons can satisfy the standards. Persons affected by chronic limitations, and especially those in the long-term-care network, are among the most likely to be overlooked or even purposely excluded. An alternative perspective to the social comparison model is achievable by defining the criteria used for successful aging relative to each person's current health status and living arrangements. In essence, the emphasis in this model is on optimizing a person's success at aging given their current situation, rather than meeting predetermined criteria of successful aging that are applied to the whole population.

The Premises of Our Research

There were two basic premises for our research. First, the range of definitions for successful aging or success at aging should allow even people with multiple illnesses and functional impairments to have the possibility of being classified as aging successfully. Second, the term *successful aging* or *success at aging* should *not* imply that some older persons will be automatically labeled as "aging unsuccessfully." We appreciate the positive connotations that often accompany the designation of successful aging, but believe it is neither necessary nor justified to label as unsuccessful anyone who is among the survivors of their birth cohort. There is, however, no reason to think that any individual researcher or author intends to label anyone as aging unsuccessfully. The risk of such a label is more likely to arise almost by default if the literature has focused heavily on select populations and exclusive definitions of successful aging.

One perspective on successful aging that appears to have especially good potential, by being sufficiently flexible to accommodate the trajectories of specific individuals, is the concept of "selective optimization with compensation" proposed by Baltes and Baltes (1990, p. 21). In essence, this approach defines those who are successfully aging as individuals who choose to make the best use of the capacities and resources they still have, despite illness and functional problems, while also finding ways to compensate for these limitations. Although these individuals will likely have to curtail or even give up some activities, success comes from making the effort to sustain the most valued activities and to compensate for others. It is important to note that selective optimization with compensation does *not* preclude using high standards of productivity and sustained vitality in the definition of success. However, it also allows for expanding the definition to include other indicators that are less ambitious. In fact, Baltes and Baltes (1990a) and an additional article by M. Baltes (1994) presented examples of promoting successful aging based on the design of a nursing home environment—certainly a setting that is characterized by persons with significant health problems. Similarly, Smyer (1995) discussed successful aging in continuing-care retirement communities, a setting designed to allow residential transitions and aging in place despite any changes in health status.

The concept of selective optimization with compensation that was advanced by Baltes and Baltes (1990a) is complemented by Rowe and Kahn's discussion of successful aging (1997, 1998), in the context of the MacArthur Foundation Research Network on Successful Aging. Rowe and Kahn described successful aging as having three components: the *physical dimension* of avoiding disease, the *psychological dimension* of maintaining high cognitive and physical function, and the *social dimension* of being engaged with life. The inclusion of social engagement as a component of successful aging is significant and appropriately reflects results of research showing the association between psychosocial variables and health status. In the presence of physical and psychological decline, two elements of Rowe and Kahn's framework, social engagement and reciprocity, are resources that can continue to foster successful aging. It is therefore important to determine how these activities are continued and encouraged in a residential setting such as assisted living.

Finally, another reason for conducting this investigation was that reports about successful aging have often been based on secondary analysis of existing information. That is, the data were originally collected to examine other topics related to aspects of life in older age (e.g., continued employment after age 65, volunteer work, functional health status) but were later often reanalyzed or interpreted under the rubric of successful aging. In these reanalyses, successful aging has sometimes been defined by longevity or simply by sustained good health. As a result, inferences about successful aging have often been made a posteriori to the original study, rather than being based on data collected for the a priori purpose of examining success at aging, including informing participants of that purpose when they were recruited. The MacArthur Research Network on Successful Aging is an important exception, but it did not focus on older persons living in congregate living arrangements.

Reciprocity and Successful Aging

The role of social support as a factor in the health and broader quality of life of older persons has been established over many years of research (e.g., Institute of Medicine, 1990; Kahn, 1994). Although much of the social support and social network research in aging has emphasized the benefits *to* the older person, there has also been attention to older adults as givers and to the reciprocal exchanges that occur between older people, their family and friends, and the broader community. These discussions can be found in long-standing literature in gerontology on the topics of friendships in older adulthood, grandparenthood, the desire to leave a legacy to one's family, volunteerism, and the concept of a social network "convoy" who pass through aging together and provide mutual support (Ingersoll-Dayton & Antonucci, 1988; Kahn & Antonucci, 1980; Litwin, 1998; Rook, 1987; Wentowski, 1981). Even the authors of the substantial literature on caregiving of older adults have considered the perspective of the older person as a care-provider or contributor to others, despite also receiving assistance (Dunkle, 1985; Krause, Herzog, & Baker, 1992; Pruchno, Burant, & Peters, 1997). There is consensus among researchers and clinicians that making contributions or feeling useful has a positive effect on life satisfaction of the older care-receiver. However, the research on care-giving and care-receiving does not appear to have looked explicitly at the exchange process in the broader framework of successful aging.

There is also an empirical and conceptual foundation from which to begin an investigation of reciprocity. For more than 20 years an area of study in the sociology of aging has dealt with what is commonly called "exchange theory" (Dowd, 1975, 1980). This literature includes the notion of reciprocity (Horwitz, Reinhard, & Howell-White, 1996; Jones & Vaughan, 1990; McCulloch, 1990). In this literature, however, reciprocity is most often conceptualized as the degree of equality or balance of exchanges between individuals and groups—a perspective akin to maintaining a ledger book of giving and receiving, and judging the quality of relationships accordingly. We did not use this balance-sheet type of reciprocity. It is entirely possible, of course, that the need to give for each act of receiving, or to receive for each act of giving, is one of the definitions used by some people. However, reciprocity can also include what has been called nonreciprocal or unbalanced exchanges (Ingersoll-Dayton & Antonucci, 1988), as well as what Wentowski (1981) termed "generalized reciprocity"—giving to others or the community at large (such as in preparing foods for bake sales, donating to charities, giving gifts spontaneously) where the contribution by the older person is not in return for a specific prior favor, or to mark an event such as a birthday.

The importance of reciprocity or contributing to others has been recognized in the literature on successful aging. As noted above, Rowe and Kahn (1997, 1998) cite social engagement as one of the three foundations of successful aging. Featherman, Smith, and Peterson (1990) discussed successful aging in the context of transactions or exchange between the person and their environment (pp. 53, 77). Both groups of authors have also contributed the notion that resilience, the ability to bounce back after an adverse event, can be a facet of successful aging, one which can be influenced by the quality of one's social network relationships. It is also the case, however, that the successful-aging literature has defined social engagement and reciprocity as the a priori markers of success, rather than investigating the degree to which they contribute to a person's perception of success (e.g., Vaillant, 1994). That is, social engagement and reciprocity have been treated as sufficient outcomes to indicate success, not as means or avenues to achieve success at aging defined by other, perhaps broader criteria. We believe that the former perspective on reciprocity is legitimate, but not complete; therefore, our project examined reciprocity as a correlate of perceived success at aging. We selected several privately owned residential assisted living facilities as the setting for our investigation.

Assisted Living as a Research Context

Assisted living (also referred to as residential care or personal care) has developed as an alternative to nursing home care for older adults who need personal assistance but do not require the amount of skilled medical care provided in nursing homes. Assisted living is a rather recent, increasingly popular form of long-term care defined as "a program that provides and/or arranges for the provision of daily meals, personal and other supportive services, health care and 24–hour oversight to persons residing in a group residential facility who need assistance with activities of daily living" (American Association of Homes and Services for the Aging, 1999). Lasky (1999) described the goal of assisted living as being "to satisfy consumers' desire to 'age in place' as long as possible in a safe, residential environment." Considering both licensed and unlicensed settings, these assisted living and personal care facilities have become a significant component of the long-term-care system (Spector, Reschovsky, & Cohen, 1996). It is now estimated that more than 1 million older adults live in an estimated 20,000 assisted living residences in the United States (Assisted Living Federation of America, 2002), and 38 state Medicaid programs provide some reimbursement for assisted living services (Mollica, 2000). Growth in the assisted living industry has been driven by consumer demand for residential options other than nursing homes and by government interest in assisted living placements as lower cost alternatives to nursing homes care.

Assisted living settings are an important context in which to investigate successful aging. The average elderly resident of an assisted living facility is female, 80 years of age, ambulatory, and needs assistance with approximately two activities of daily living (Kraditor, 2001). The reasons individuals and older couples have for making a move to assisted living can have significant implications for their perceptions of success at aging, as well as for the options they have for sustaining reciprocity. Typically, the move to assisted living is made due to existing health problems or to concern about susceptibility to potentially serious problems. After years of independence and living in a home or apartment, making a residential move can challenge an individual's assessments of how their aging has proceeded and their expectations for the future. The day-to-day experiences of being in the assisted living residence can therefore have a substantial impact on the way individuals resolve the fundamental questions of dependence versus competence, and the degree to which they feel they are successfully dealing with their aging. The design of the living environment, the delivery of services within the facility, and perhaps even staff-resident interactions can foster the objectives of optimizing competence and success at aging.

Research Questions

With this background in mind, our project was designed to interview residents and staff at assisted living settings on the topics of successful aging and reciprocity. The following questions guided the project:

1. What standards or criteria do older adults living in assisted living facilities use to define successful aging?
2. Is reciprocity correlated with individuals' assessments of their successful aging?
3. What is the potential for assisted living settings to promote the reciprocity of residents, and thereby contribute to their successful aging or success at aging?

Data Collection

All data for this project were collected at residential sites owned by a private corporation that operates catered retirement living and assisted living facilities in Rhode Island, southeastern Massachusetts, and Connecticut. Our project was conducted at four sites in proximity to Brown University. The residences have a gracious style with amenities of various types at the sites (e.g., large entrance lobbies, spacious dining rooms with vaulted ceilings, on-site meal preparation and wait staff, ice cream parlors with sitting areas, pubs with pool tables, an exercise room, hairdressing room, library with computer access, a private dining room for resident-reserved functions, large common room with television, on-site health care staff, and local transportation). All sites had an activities director and were built specifically for the services they provide. The oldest residence had been built about 9 years before we began this research project in January 2000.

These characteristics of the residences are the background against which this project must be placed. As with any research, the findings of our project are conditional upon those who volunteered to participate. In this regard, the residential settings that permitted us to recruit residents appeared to be about as supportive of the project as could be hoped for, as were the residents themselves.

Pilot Phase: Months 1–6

We used the first 6 months of the project for interview development and pilot testing. Phase 1 provided experience in asking questions about successful aging and reciprocity, because relatively little research had queried older adults directly, as noted before. We tested interview questions with 24 residents, 4 of whom were men. Several of the interview questions were used to obtain specific examples of successful aging and reciprocity, which became the basis for predefined lists during the main phase of data collection described below.

We used a single residential facility for the pilot test. We did not want to have mailings and formal meetings with the residents at all of the residences for the pilot test and again for the main phase of data collection. Given the daily flow of events at a residence, it did not seem practical to make detailed contacts and presentations at all sites, then wait several months to recontact persons for the main phase of data collection in months 7 through 12.

Main Phase: Months 7–12

Resident Interview

Interviews with the residents for the main study began with obtaining general background information, including their current health problems. This was followed by a gait speed assessment that timed the participant on two walks over a 10–meter distance (we averaged the times and converted them to meters/seconds walked). The next portion of the interview was on reciprocity and was followed by the section on successful aging and a few more general background questions. After this content was collected, we administered three questionnaires designed to assess psychosocial status: Philadelphia Geriatric Center Morale Scale (PGC), Life Satisfaction Index-A (LSIA), and the MHI-5

indicator of recent mood status from the Medical Outcomes Study).
These three instruments were chosen in order to examine whether
any associations observed between perceived successful aging and reciprocity might be empirically explained as primarily representing more
general life satisfaction and perceived well-being.

Successful Aging and Reciprocity. Three methods were used to assess success at aging and reciprocity. The interview questions were parallel for
both topics, although the wording was specific to each. The first question presented a predefined list of ways that persons might have successful aging and might give to or receive from others. Participants
were given printed lists of the options as an aid to answering. Multiple
answers were allowed, and participants also could add other ways of
having successful aging, or giving and receiving. The items in the list
were generated from the interviews conducted during months 1
through 6, when participants were asked to provide examples of successful aging and reciprocity.

The second method was a self-anchored ladder rating scale. We
asked participants to rate their overall success at aging and ability to
give to or help others on a scale of 0 (worst possible) through 10 (best
possible). We asked for past, present, and future ratings, and also for
a description of why they chose a particular rating for each time point.
The past rating was for 1 year prior to moving into the residence, and the
future rating was for 2 years hence. If participants rated themselves currently as less than a 9 or 10, the interviewer asked if there were any
specific activities or circumstances that might raise them to that level.

Third, the sections on reciprocity and successful aging each included a set of Likert-type items designed by the research team. The intent
of these items was to pilot a possible scale for assessing older adults'
overall judgments of their current reciprocity and their current success at aging. In contrast to the ladder ratings, they were not anchored
with perceived best and worst situations. The wording of the statements was purposely kept general and not tied to specific examples of
reciprocity or successful aging (i.e., such as appeared in the lists that
were given in the interview). These items were an experimental part
of the project, but having them in the interview seemed to be promising given the dearth of measures available to even estimate older
persons' own perceptions of their status in these two areas.

The two sets of Likert-type questions (for successful aging and for
reciprocity) were structured similarly. First, participants selected one of
three "stem" statements that they felt best represented their feelings about

reciprocity and about successful aging: (1) I feel that I am not [having very much success at aging/doing well at giving to others] at the current time; (2) I feel that I am doing as well as can be expected [having success at aging/giving to others]; (3) I feel that I am [having very good success at aging/doing very well with giving to others]. Number 1 represented a negative response, and numbers 2 and 3 represented a positive response. Based on a positive or negative response to the stem question, the interviewer then read a series of statements (about reciprocity and successful aging, respectively), and asked participants to agree or disagree with each one according to the Likert method (agree a lot, agree a little, neither agree nor disagree, disagree a little, disagree a lot). The statements following a negative stem response were not worded exactly the same as those that followed a positive stem response. For example, "I am less successful in my older age than other people I know," "I lose more than I gain by trying to be successful in my older age," "It is important for me to feel successful in my older age," and "I feel more successful at aging than I expected to feel at my current age." This approach is somewhat novel in the design of a psychosocial assessment scale. However, our thought was that a negative response to the stem question placed the individual in a different context than did a positive response and could therefore require some different follow-up items rather than using a single set of items.

Background Information. The background information about each resident included demographics of age, gender, race, education, social networks (e.g., number of living children and frequency of contact, proximity of any children or close relatives or friends to the residence), and health status (e.g., current health problems or conditions, number of medications, number of hospital and doctor visits, ability to perform activities of daily living, use of a cane or walker). We also asked about their reasons for moving to the residence, how frequently they left the residence, and their mode of transportation.

Qualitative Questions. There were also questions in the interview that were intended to be more qualitative in nature and had open-ended responses. These included: Are there things the administrators and staff of the residence can do to help you [have a successful older age/do things for others]? Is there anything that you would like to do for family, friends, or people in the community that you do not currently do here at the residence? If you were to give advice to younger people, in their 30's, 40's, and 50's, about how to be successful in older age, what would you say?

Staff Interview

The staff interview began with a background section, asking for the respondent's age, gender, race, and information about their job, such as length of time in their current position, job responsibilities, certification (if applicable), and usual shift. These questions were followed by a section to assess opinions about reciprocity, and then a section to assess opinions about successful aging.

Both the successful aging and reciprocity portions of the staff interview asked for examples of ways in which residents showed the concept being addressed (i.e., reciprocity or successful aging). There were then three additional open-ended questions: How does the residence and staff help the residents do things for others/have a successful older age? In your own interactions with the residents, how do you encourage the residents to do things for others/ enhance their success at aging? In your own interactions, how could you do more, with adequate time and resources? Finally, there was an event sampling question that asked for three specific instances in which the respondent or other staff helped a resident to contribute to others/promote their successful aging.

Interview Sample

We completed a total of 88 resident interviews and 42 staff interviews at six residences. The resident interviews ranged from 45 to 90 minutes and usually took place in the resident's apartment. We scheduled the interview to accommodate the participant's best time, with most taking place in the morning or midafternoon. Staff interviews, which took only 10 to 15 minutes, occurred during the workday at a time convenient for the staff member.

Resident Characteristics

Characteristics of the residents are shown in Table 2.1. As expected, the majority were women, although just over 25% were men. Average age was 82.8 (SD = 5.96; range = 68–93). All participants described themselves as Caucasian non-Hispanic, and the majority (96%) said that their incomes were adequate to meet their needs. These latter two characteristics of the sample should be kept in mind when considering results of the interviews.

The project team went to each setting in advance and held a session (advertised by letter and in the residence newspaper) to present the project, answer questions, and begin the recruitment process. Individ-

Table 2.1 Selected Characteristics of Residents Who Were Interviewed

Characteristic	Number	Percentage
Gender:		
Female	64	72.7
Male	24	27.3
Marital status:		
Married	23	26.1
All other	65	73.9
Formal education:		
Less than HS	8	9.1
High/Trade school	35	39.8
Some college	14	15.9
College grad	21	23.9
Post-graduate	10	11.4
Age group:		
68–79	22	25.0
80–85	33	37.5
86–93	33	37.5
Time at residence:		
Less than 1 year	18	20.5
1 year–18 months	30	34.1
19 months–2 years	24	27.3
More than 2 years	16	18.2
Self-rated health		
Excellent/Very Good	19	22.1
Good	34	39.5
Fair/Poor	33	38.4

uals could volunteer at that time or make contact afterwards. Interviews at each setting were carried out over at least a 1-month period.

Participation was not equal across the settings: residence 1 = 36; residence 2 = 16; residence 3 = 11; residence 4 = 0; residence 5 = 16, and residence 6 = 11. Two of the four sites had two separate residences, so we considered them to have two residences each. Our experience was that the overall health status of residents and the internal support by the on-site administration were key factors in generating participation. All sites had residents of advanced age with chronic health problems, but some sites appeared to have relatively more limited residents. Also, the sites differed in the degree to which the activity director and on-site administrator seemed to be receptive to the

project. Highest participation was at the site where the activity director was reported by everyone (and confirmed by our experience) to
be extremely involved with the residents, who had enthusiastic contact
with us prior to the visit, and the residents who came to the group
meeting were clearly the most functionally independent. Lowest participation (no interviewees, despite some attendance at the presentation) was at the site where the activity director said she had not read
our introductory materials in any detail and tried to do a door-to-door
announcement the day we came to make the presentation.

Staff Characteristics

A total of 42 staff and administrators were interviewed, between 9 and
12 individuals at each of the four residential facilities. Respondents
represented all sectors of the residences: on-site management, nursing
services, personal care assistants, social/recreational activities, maintenance, and food services. The large majority ($n = 38$, 90.5%) worked
the day shift, most were women ($n = 35$, 83.3%), and virtually all were
Caucasian non-Hispanic ($n = 40$, 95.2%). Exactly half ($n = 21$) said
they had a professional license or certification.

The average ages across the four settings were: 37.7 ($SD = 13.7$),
39.5 ($SD = 16.4$), 43.2 ($SD = 13.8$), and 45.3 ($SD = 8.9$). Time worked
at the residence ranged from 3 months to 10 years, with average times
across the four settings of 14.9 months, 17.2 months, 34.0 months,
and 37.6 months. In addition, 62% of the staff ($n = 26$) said that they
had worked in other assisted living, congregate care, or nursing home
facilities, and for those who did, the average time was just over 10
years, with a range of 14 months to 35 years.

Results

Research Question 1: What Standards or Criteria Are Used to Define Successful Aging?

Results from the Predefined List

Table 2.2 presents the criteria that respondents stated they used to
judge whether or not they were aging successfully, based on the responses to the interview question that gave them the predefined list of

Table 2.2 Participants' Reports of Ways to Have Success at Aging
(*n* = 88)

Characteristic	Number	Percentage
Staying active	57	64.8
Be proud of family/children	54	61.4
Keeping in touch with others	52	59.1
Keeping a positive outlook	48	54.5
Maintaining health	47	53.4
Being friendly/outgoing	47	53.4
Keeping hobbies/interests	44	50.0
Having good friends	41	46.6
Coping well with changes	34	38.6
Can still drive oneself	28	31.8
Being a volunteer	26	29.5
Looking good for one's age	25	28.4
Still able to travel	22	25.0
Receiving compliments	18	20.5
Recovering from illness	17	19.3
Being asked for advice	14	15.9
Living to a certain age	13	14.8
Starting new hobbies/interests	11	12.5
Working for pay	5	5.7
Being told they are right	3	3.4

options. Table 2.2 is organized in decreasing order of prevalence, but placement in the *list* was not associated with the percentage of endorsement. For example, one of the lowest percentages occurred for the first item in the list (still working for pay), and the highest percentage came in the middle of the list (keeping active).

There was clearly a wide range of endorsements to the items in the list, but because of the size of our sample one should not take the rank ordering too literally. However, Table 2.2 does suggest that a variety of circumstances can be perceived as contributing to a feeling of successful aging, and we do not yet want to dismiss any items in the list as unimportant.

Respondents also had the option to add other answers to the standard list, and those responses were entered into the NVivo qualitative data management package (QSR, 2000). In some instances, the responses offered here were restatements of items on the predefined list but still merit mentioning because of their probable importance as keyword designations of older adults' perspectives, rather than investigator-designated labels. The following were offered as ways to judge how successfully one was aging: being independent, including financially independent; not defining oneself as old; retaining faith and spirituality; feeling good about oneself, and doing things for others to make them feel good/happy.

Ladder Ratings

Table 2.3 presents the results for the three ladder ratings for successful aging: Current, 1 year prior to entering the residence, and 2 years into the future.

The table indicates that a lower percentage of respondents placed themselves in the highest successful aging categories (9–10) currently, relative to the year before they moved to the residence. Although our sample was comprised of volunteers, it is evident and of equal importance that the participants were not exclusively those who believed they were having optimal success at aging.

One other trend to note in the results shown in Table 2.3 is that the percentage in the lowest category increases and the percentage in the highest category decreases. The increase in the lowest category is attributable to the higher number of respondents who gave a "don't know" response to the 2-Year-Future Ladder rating—a total of 35 participants. The higher prevalence of "don't know" answers to the future-oriented ladder is consistent with findings from Rakowski's research on the topic of older adults' future time perspective. In that research, don't knows tended to have the same associations with other variables as did an explicit response of having a limited future time perspective.

Table 2.3 Ratings for Self-Perceived Successful Aging Using the Ladder Methodology

Rating on the ladder	Time frame for the rating		
	1–Year premove (%)	Current (%)	2–Year future (%)
0–4/Don't Know	14.1	5.9	48.8
5–6	9.4	17.6	11.3
7	4.7	8.7	1.3
8	16.5	32.9	21.3
9–10	55.3	35.3	17.5

We therefore classified "don't know" answers in the least favorable category.

Likert-Item Indices

These were the sets of items answered on a strongly agree/disagree scale. The possible range for each scale was 1.00 (*lowest/most unfavorable*) to 5.00 (*highest/most favorable*). The scales had the following characteristics: *Successful Aging Index: M* = 3.53, *SD* = .66; *Reciprocity Index: M* = 3.64, *SD* = .80

Similar to the results for the ladder rating, the mean values show that not all of our respondents believed they were at the optimal point of reciprocity and experiencing successful aging. The values also suggest that there was not a bias towards agreement in a direction presumed to be desirable.

Qualitative Responses

There were two qualitative items in the interview that could also provide examples of successful aging. One of these was follow-up after the Current Ladder ratings, when persons who did not rate themselves a 9 or 10 were asked what activities or circumstances might raise them to that level. The second was an open-ended question about the advice they would give to younger adults in order to have success at aging. These responses were organized using NVivo, and mirrored those given to the entries in the redefined list (Table 2.2).

Current Ladder Rating. Independence and physical health were cited often, with mobility within the residence and the ability to drive also being reported. Helping others and social contact were also mentioned. Otherwise, there was just a smattering of other replies (e.g., requests for more intellectual stimulation and more exercise programs). In fact, several residents explicitly stated that it would not be possible to reach the level of a 9–10.

Advice to Younger Persons. The majority of participants were able to offer some advice; very few said they had nothing to recommend. The most frequent types of advice fell into the categories of maintaining health and good habits; helping others and the community; planning for and having financial independence into one's older age; staying active and having outside interests; having a social network; keeping a positive outlook and enjoying each day, and staying flexible when dealing with life changes. Setting goals and working to achieve them was evident in many responses. Mentioned less often were maintaining spirituality and having solid personal values.

Research Question 2: Is Reciprocity Associated With Individuals' Assessments of Successful Aging?

Bivariate Correlations Between Successful Aging and Reciprocity

Table 2.4 shows the zero-order correlations between successful aging and reciprocity. The table includes both the Ladder and Likert versions of the indices for successful aging and for reciprocity, as well as the Current and Future orientation of the indices.

The Current Reciprocity Ladder rating was significantly correlated with the Current Successful Aging Ladder ($r = .36$; $p < .001$), and the Current Reciprocity Likert index was significantly associated with the Current Successful Aging Likert index ($r = .59$; $p < .001$). In addition, the Future Reciprocity Ladder was significantly correlated with the Future Successful Aging Ladder ($r = .56$, $p < .001$). Although these are only bivariate associations, they indicated an association between the two constructs.

In addition, two other points are worth noting. First, the two Current Successful Aging indicators are only moderately correlated ($r =$

Table 2.4 Bivariate Correlations Between Successful Aging and Reciprocity

	Current	Current		Future	
	Reciprocity: Likert	Success: Ladder	Success: Likert	Reciprocity: Ladder	Success: Ladder
Current:					
Reciprocity: Ladder	.43	.36	.29	.50	.27
Reciprocity: Likert	—	.39	.59	.36	.24
Current:					
Success: Ladder		—	.45	.28	.46
Success: Likert			—	.38	.37
Future:					
Reciprocity: Ladder				—	.56

.45; $p < .001$), as are the two Current Reciprocity indicators ($r = .43$; $p < .001$). We cannot say, at this time, whether this moderate level correlation, although still statistically significant, means that one indicator is more valid than the other or that each indicator comes at the targeted construct from somewhat different perspectives. However, the results of the regression analyses (presented below) lead us to conclude that it is prudent, for the time being, to consider them different ways of estimating the construct being assessed.

Second, the correlation between the Current Reciprocity Likert index and the Current Successful Aging Ladder is significant ($r = .36$; $p < .001$), as is the correlation between the Current Reciprocity Ladder and the Current Successful Aging Likert index ($r = .29$; $p < .008$). These correlations represent cross-method estimates of association between the two constructs, given that one is based on the Ladder rating and the other is based on the multi-item index. These correlations are slightly lower than those based on the same method. It is therefore possible that a modest degree of response-set exists for the Ladder rating method and the Likert-type method, which acts to boost the intramethod correlations. However, the presence of these significant cross-method correlations supports the inference that the two constructs are in fact associated.

Multiple Regression Analyses

Multiple regression analyses were conducted, using successful aging as the dependent variable. There were three dependent variables in these analyses. We used the Current Ladder rating and the multi-item Likert-scale index as indicators of current perceived successful aging, and the 2–Year Future Ladder ratings as the third dependent variable. (These results are shown in Tables 2.5, 2.6, and 2.7.)

Due to the small sample size of residents, it was important to avoid having too many independent variables in the analysis. We first examined bivariate associations by computing correlations or analyses of variance (as appropriate). Also, we were careful to avoid including covariates in the multiple regression analyses that were themselves associated at .40 or above, to limit the risk of colinearity. Therefore, the analyses shown here are based on our best judgment of the most appropriate covariates based on the bivariate associations.

As a part of the examination of bivariate associations, we calculated an average score for the LSIA and for the three subscales of the PGC Morale Scale (Agitation, Attitudes Toward Own Aging, Lonely Dissatisfaction). Bivariate associations showed that the PGC Agitation subscale was not strongly related to successful aging, but that the Attitudes Toward Own Aging and Lonely Dissatisfaction subscales were associated. We therefore calculated an average score based on the combined items for these latter two subscales. This combined average score was more strongly associated with successful aging than was the LSIA scale. Because the LSIA and the averaged PGC subscore correlated at a prohibitively high .67, we decided to use only the combined PGC subscore in the regression analyses. This is referred to as the PGC Composite index when presenting the results.

Analyses for Current Successful Aging. Table 2.5 shows the results of analyses for the Ladder rating of current successful aging, and Table 2.6 shows the results for the Likert index of current successful aging.

Due to the nature of our sample, we prefer to look at the analyses for current perceived successful aging as a whole, rather than propose a best indicator of successful aging or try to identify only the best covariates across all analyses. From this perspective, perceptions of successful aging were associated with better perceived reciprocity, gender (i.e., being female), having lived a longer time at the residence, and having more favorable scores on the PGC composite index.

Two points are worth noting about these results. First, it is not surprising that the PGC composite was associated with perceived successful aging, because the two variables would each be expected to reflect an assessment of the quality of one's life. However, the PGC composite did not overwhelm perceived reciprocity (in a statistical sense), suggesting that the association between reciprocity and suc-

Table 2.5 Results of Multiple Regression Analysis of the Ladder Rating for Current Successful Aging

Covariate	beta weight	SE	t-score	p-value
Reciprocity ladder	.14	.08	1.73	.087
PGC composite	2.09	.49	4.31	< .001
Time lived at residence	.44	.11	4.06	< .001
Gender	−.76	.23	−3.29	.002
Gait speed	.17	.13	1.28	.204

Note: Multiple R = .699; Multiple R^2 = .489; Adjusted Multiple R^2 = .453; F = 13.77; N = 78; $p < .0001$.

Table 2.6 Results of Multiple Regression Analysis of the Likert Index of Current Successful Aging

Covariate	beta weight	SE	t-score	p-value
Reciprocity index	.33	.09	3.81	< .001
PGC composite	.79	.34	2.36	.021
Total health problems	−.03	.03	−1.27	.208
Age	−.01	.01	−.58	.563
Gait speed	−.05	.08	−.59	.559
MHI-5	.11	.20	.54	.589
Self-rated health	.04	.09	.43	.665
How often leaves residence	.12	.17	.71	.482

Note: Multiple R = .726; Multiple R^2 = .527; Adjusted Multiple R^2 = .469; F = 9.06; N = 74; p < .0001.

cessful aging might in fact be robust. (*Note:* Without the PGC composite score in the regression, reciprocity was associated with the Ladder rating of successful aging at p < .002 and with the Likert index at p < .001.)

The second point is that many other potential covariates were not associated with successful aging, nor did the total number of health problems statistically overwhelm perceived reciprocity as a covariate. Several potential covariates (e.g., education, marital status, recency of seeing children or others) did not show strong enough bivariate associations to be included in the regressions, and those that were included did not eliminate the association of reciprocity with successful aging. Again, our sample was small, which introduces the possibility of biases, nuances, or artifacts in the correlation matrices upon which the regressions are based, which might have operated in favor of the reciprocity/ successful aging association. Clearly, there is need for additional data, but the results for now are encouraging.

Analysis for Future Successful Aging. Table 2.7 shows the results of analyses for the Ladder rating of future successful aging.

There was a surprising lack of covariates for the Ladder rating of 2-year future success at aging. The majority of covariates that had bivariate associations did not emerge as significant in the multiple regression analyses. The Ladder rating for current successful aging was used as a covariate for statistical control, on the premise that baseline perceived

Table 2.7 Results of Multiple Regression Analysis of the Ladder Rating of Future Successful Aging

Covariate	beta weight	SE	t-score	p-value
Reciprocity ladder.	.48	.12	3.99	.002
Successful aging ladder	.43	.14	3.12	.003
Able to drive oneself	.64	.34	1.90	.062
ER visit in past year	−.37	.33	−1.15	.256
Total health problems	−.05	.07	−.70	.487
Age	−.04	.03	−1.31	.194
MD visits/past year	−.09	.18	−.48	.633
Gait speed	−.01	.22	−.03	.973
PGC composite	−.30	.82	−.37	.716

Note: Multiple R = .723; Multiple R^2 = .522; Adjusted Multiple R^2 = .452; F = 7.41; N = 71; p < .0001.

successful aging would be a strong correlate of expected future successful aging. That premise was supported. The only other statistically significant correlate was the Ladder rating for 2-year future reciprocity, again suggesting an association between the two concepts.

The trend for being able to drive a car also merits attention. The capacity to drive oneself was cited by a few participants in the open-ended questions as an important piece of evidence of their sustained abilities, which has been noted in the overall gerontological literature for many years. The inability to drive is a serious challenge to one's sense of independence and a source of concern about vulnerability.

Research Question 3: What Is the Potential for Assisted Living Settings to Promote Successful Aging?

In retrospect, this turned out to be the least quantifiable of the specific aims because it relied on the responses of the residents and the staff members to direct questions about what residence staff and the facility as a whole might do to support successful aging and reciprocity.

Successful Aging: Resident Responses

Slightly more than half of the sample (n = 51) stated that they did not think residence staff and management could do more to promote their successful aging. We could not determine the degree to which this percentage is a function of a facilitative environment that already exists at the residence, or a perception of the residents that it is not the responsibility of staff or management, or an assessment that their successful aging cannot be substantially enhanced, or a reluctance of residents to sound critical of the residence and management given their dependence on the residence (despite our comments during recruitment that we were funded independently and would not share individuals' comments with administrators). Future investigations should be prepared for what may seem like a high percentage of participants who see no potential in their residence, and follow-up questions should be prepared to pursue the topic to assess reasons.

Of those who offered an answer, responses fell into the categories of providing additional services, adding more intellectually stimulating activities, allowing unscheduled events and activities that arise from resident initiative, involving residents in event planning, having more effective and involved on-site administration, hiring more staff, and improving the quality of the food.

Successful Aging: Staff Responses

When staff were asked what it meant to be successful at this stage of the residents' lives, being independent was most frequently cited ($n = 15$). Staff defined independence as the residents' having physical and mental faculties or, when these decrease, still being able to do for themselves. Several other factors noted by staff centered on a theme of engagement, such as being with people and having friends ($n = 4$), having family ($n = 1$), staying active ($n = 3$), and being useful ($n = 3$). Staff felt they helped residents to be successful in their older age, despite health problems, by engaging residents in activities ($n = 16$). Staff cited the offering of activities as well as the encouragement of residents to participate in the activities offered. The theme of encouragement surfaced through other comments relating to bolstering residents' self-esteem, (that is, making them feel important ($n = 8$) and encouraging independence through verbal prompting and staff actions ($n = 7$). Two staff respondents felt that nothing in particular was done to promote residents' successful aging.

Staff felt that with adequate time and resources they could further promote residents' successful aging by being nice to them; that is, by spending more time with residents ($n = 18$) and by the facilities' offering more activities and more diverse activities and services ($n = 20$).

Staff who cited more diversity in activities and services ($n = 8$) as a way to promote successful aging gave as examples gardening, animal and music programs, massage, and psychosocial services (i.e., social services and support groups). More family involvement ($n = 4$), opportunities to volunteer or to use volunteers, such as an intergenerational program ($n = 3$), outings ($n = 3$), physical activities ($n = 3$), and personalized activities ($n = 3$) were some proposed activity enhancements. Seven staff members either did not know what else could be done or felt that staff "can't do much more."

Conclusions

Successful aging and reciprocity were meaningful concepts to at least a subgroup of people who lived at the residences. They attended our initial presentation, which was straightforward about the topics to be studied (we distributed the interview for review), and decided the topics had enough merit to participate. People were able to provide examples of successful aging and reciprocity, and endorsed items in the predefined lists that were presented during the interview (Table 2.2). It is worth noting that not everyone who was interviewed endorsed a high level of successful aging (or reciprocity), so there was variance on the measures used in the analyses. Our data did not appear to be affected by a bias to agree with high degrees of current or future successful aging and reciprocity.

In addition, the regression analyses indicated that reciprocity and successful aging had an empirically robust association. This result supports the premises in the literature on successful aging and social support, as well as a report by Fisher (1995) that qualitatively examined the meaning of successful aging in a small sample of older persons and found an association with perceptions of contributing to others. In addition, a more general marker of life satisfaction (the PGC composite) did not eliminate the association between reciprocity and perceived successful aging. Had the PGC composite score been the dominant correlate, this would have suggested that perceived successful aging might well simply reflect a more general perception about the quality of life.

One of the important implications from our project is the need for administrators and staff always to be aware that the little things and interpersonal niceties of day-to-day life have a substantial impact on residents' assessments of the quality of their lives. This is consistent with the theme of everyday activities discussed by Horgas, Wilms, and Baltes (1998) and the concept of every day competence discussed by Diehl (1998) and by Wahl, Oswald, and Zimprich (1999). Ryff (1989) proposed six fundamental areas of successful aging: self-acceptance, positive relations with others, autonomy, environmental mastery, purpose in life, and personal growth. These general themes are relevant to daily life in an assisted living facility, even if the congregate nature of the setting requires adapting these six areas to the context. Ryff also highlighted the importance of asking older adults for their own criteria for successful aging.

The point to emphasize is that there are probably very few features of an assisted living setting that are too small to overlook as opportunities to benefit residents. It is unrealistic to expect being able to involve (or please) all residents all of the time, or maybe even most residents most of the time; and there are undoubtedly limits to what the facilities can provide without charging excessive fees. However, we feel safe inferring from our results that resources put into staff training, activities planning, providing volunteer opportunities, and encouraging what might simply be described as being nice to each other on a daily basis will reap large rewards for residents' assessments of how they are aging. These recommendations may not seem that ambitious relative to the images of high-achieving elders that are used in the media to market products, but they appear to be an important and necessary foundation for promotion of successful aging.

Beyond having a solid infrastructure at the residence, there is another consideration: Some of our sample cited a desire for more intellectually stimulating activities in order to optimize successful aging. Assisted living facilities should be alert for the residents who want these options. We did not pursue their answers to identify the specific activities or resources they desired; in hindsight, it may well be a response we should have anticipated and been prepared to follow up. The residences each posted their monthly activity calendars, and our impression was that the days were always full, including off-site activities. Our recommendation at this point is simply that the administration and staff of assisted living residences have a periodic review of the content of their activities calendar from the perspective of what might be described as intellectual challenges. The literature on aging repeatedly sensitizes us to the diversity of the older population and the life histories that evolve as people age. There is every reason to expect that this diversity (and correspondingly diverse interests) will be reflected in the clientele of assisted living settings.

We are encouraged that further research can be conducted in assisted living facilities, and our project will hopefully be one of many that examine successful aging in special populations, such as persons with HIV/AIDS as was described by Kahana and Kahana (2001); the examination of lay theories of successful aging among recent widows conducted by Bergstrom and Holmes (2000); and a report on perceptions of successful aging among nursing home residents by Guse and Masesar (1999). However, there are some points to keep in mind as more work is done in assisted living settings. First, participation by residents was not as good as we had hoped. No more than 40% of the attendees at any of the presentations signed up for the interview. It was hard to generate broad enthusiasm, and it was background work by the activity director before and after the informational presentation that made a big difference in recruiting residents. We have no basis therefore on which to make estimates of the percentage of persons in this type of residential setting who believe they are (or are not) having success at aging or who are having a gratifying reciprocal association with their social and residential environment.

Second, the residences used in this research are at the upper end of current assisted-living settings. Residents can afford individual apartments on a self-pay basis; and much to their credit, the corporation owners and administrators clearly place a priority on keeping a well-maintained environment, with ample social spaces and high ceilings to create a spacious atmosphere. Our impression is that if two somewhat abstract (or ideal) concepts like successful aging and reciprocity are going to be meaningful to very old persons in a congregate living environment, then the data will be most favorable at residences like these. Assisted living covers a diverse range of settings, not all of which are as comfortable as those in which we interviewed, nor do residents have as many capital resources on which to draw.

Therefore, it is important to broaden the type of research we have done here, to include settings that do not provide the same upscale environment and that have residents who do not have the same resources. In doing so, there will be a broader mix of racial and ethnic groups, whereas our sample was exclusively Caucasian. Our project can provide no insight on perceived successful aging and reciprocity among older adults of color.

Third, the residents were more willing to comment on current successful aging and reciprocity (i.e., the multi-item indices) and the Ladder ratings) than they were to respond to the 2-year future Ladder ratings. Almost half of the sample responded with "don't know" or refused to answer the 2-year future ratings. This is very likely a key factor in the high correlation between the two future-oriented Ladder ratings (Table 2.4). Given the average age of our sample (82.5) and the fact that they moved to the residence for specific reasons, it is not surprising that so many people were not certain about a time frame 2 years in the future. Still to be determined, however, is whether the promise of sustaining future successful aging can be an effective motivator for things such as participating in health promotion programs and making specific lifestyle changes.

Fourth, at this point, we have no way of knowing whether perceptions of successful aging have implications for the longer-term health and well-being of older persons such as those who participated in the research. Over the past two decades especially, a great deal of work has been done on psychosocial predictors of mortality and morbidity in older adulthood (e.g., self-rated health, social support, religiosity). To date, successful aging has been viewed primarily as a dependent variable or an outcome of other factors. This approach to the concept is important in its own right insofar as it reflects current quality of life. Still, there is no reason why an indicator of perceived present and future successful aging could not be investigated as a predictor of subsequent health status or other outcomes.

The question of how successful aging and reciprocity are defined by older persons in assisted residences is important. Our impression is that residents and staff see successful aging and reciprocity in what might be called the "little things" of daily life at the residences. Although a qualitative impression, our sense is that both residents and staff recognized the reality of having moved to a more protective setting. It would be hard to have any other perspective. Assisted residential settings are an important option in the long-term-care network, but even so they are still the equivalent of very pleasantly furnished and appointed dormitories. And the realities of congregate living in a context where many persons have health problems cannot be ignored. Therefore, even though successful aging seemed to be a meaningful concept for our sample, the specific examples cited were most often things that happened in routine daily life within the residences.

Fifth, the wording of our assessments of reciprocity (i.e., the ladder and Likert indices) emphasized the participant's perception of her or his role as a contributor or giver to others. We did not assess separately perceptions of the extent of receiving help or services and calculate some type of comparison measure, nor did we attempt to construct questions that requested participants' judgements of the overall balance in their lives between giving and receiving. Given the expected time constraints during an interview, we preferred to focus on the giver/contributor dimension because it has not been as widely represented in research. And given the context of the project, it seemed reasonable to assume that support services were a part of the daily environment for all of our participants. However, there is certainly a need to investigate further how reciprocity can be operationalized to best represent the meaning of the construct.

Other aspects of our results also deserve further attention. We did not directly probe with follow-up questions about the ability to drive, but several participants cited it as a factor that affected their sense of successful aging, as well as their ability to be reciprocal with others. There are, of course, good reasons why some people are no longer able to drive. However, the importance of driving is so symbolic that we wonder if it can be ignored. Creativity in activities planning could be helpful. For example, might it be possible for assisted living residences to create a symbolic sponsorship program, where (on a rotating basis) an individual resident is publicized as the honorary sponsor of a group trip off the grounds? It would take little effort to highlight the resident as the sponsor of the trip and perhaps provide a tastefully done symbol of their role, (such as a badge, a specially designed shirt, or an embossed name tag. (The Tour de France designates the overall leader with the yellow jersey, which passes from rider to rider as the lead changes and is a respected symbol.) The resident could even have a role in choosing the site of the trip. A similar strategy might also be used for on-site activities, such as during visits from outside groups.

Several residents and staff said the management of the residence and the corporate administration more generally did not encourage the type of associations that would support successful aging and reciprocity. These were a minority of the responses we obtained, but we did not expect them. Again, perhaps in hindsight we should have been prepared to pursue them. We have no way to verify the basis for this perception, but it is a facet of our qualitative responses that future research should keep in mind.

In addition, we did not ask residents directly to verbalize what the subjective anchors were for their ratings of successful aging and reciprocity, when using the ladder ratings and the Likert-based indices. Our pilot testing in months 1 through 6 indicated that interview time would be at a premium, so we had to make choices about what to ask. It is possible that the same numerical rating at two or even all three time-points could have different reference criteria. For example, recognition of the more restricted environment of a residence (compared to living independently in the community), as well as any limitations to one's health and resources, might well lead to less ambitious criteria for defining the high end of a ladder. As noted in the prior discussion, many of the specific examples that participants cited as evidence of successful aging and of reciprocity would suggest that such readjustments occur. On the one hand, changes in the criteria for reciprocity and success are not especially relevant to the fundamental question of whether older persons in assisted residential settings perceive these two concepts as still being meaningful for them. The capacity to feel successful at that point in life, and to feel like a contributor to others, is the key issue from an experiential or phenomenological perspective. It is, instructive, however, to know what the new criteria are, because it gives some insight into how older adults in assisted settings conceptualize their day-to-day life space.

Finally, from the specific examples provided for successful aging and for reciprocity there was no evidence that participants (residents or staff) were using a peer comparison standard for making their assessments. The category "looking good for my age" was about the closest to a peer comparison—which could in some instances mean looking better than others. Even this option was endorsed by only about 28% of the sample. Instead, successful aging and reciprocity were overwhelmingly based on their own personal activities. In essence, the instances cited were what a person was doing for themselves and for others, but without comparison to what others were accomplishing. There was virtually no reference to meeting or beating some standard of performance.

It would be helpful in future research to ask directly about the importance of social comparisons as a basis for one's assessment of having success at aging or having a satisfying exchange with one's social and residential environment. One of the reasons for originally proposing this research was our belief that "normative" or comparative-based standards as the definitions of successful aging and reciprocity were not sufficient. The resident and staff interviews in fact appeared to indicate that these are not the primary criteria used. It would be intriguing to ask a sample of Senior Olympics participants or the vibrant actors in television commercials about their criteria for successful aging.

Acknowledgments

The authors wish to thank Adrienne Rupp, Erica Schockett, and Laura Bonacore for their important roles in project management, interviewing, and data processing. We would also like to thank the owners of The Village Inc., as well as the on-site management and staff, for their permission to conduct the project. And a special thanks to the residents and staff who volunteered to be interviewed. This project was supported by a grant from the AARP-Andrus Foundation. Correspondence may be addressed to Dr. William Rakowski, Department of Community Health, Box G-H1, Brown University, Providence, RI 02912, USA. Or: William_Rakowski@brown.edu.

Chapter 3

Successful Aging: Intended and Unintended Consequences of a Concept

Robert L. Kahn

I n their classic book on human organizations, March and Simon (1958) emphasized the distinction between the intended and unintended consequences of bureaucratic structure. Organizations tend to gauge their success in terms of intended outcomes, such as productivity and profitability, and to ignore, or at least de-emphasize, unintended outcomes.

Both points—the importance of the distinction between intended and unintended outcomes and the almost exclusive emphasis on intended consequences—are relevant for assessing the impact of scientific concepts. Concepts, to the extent that they are influential, are likely to have effects of both kinds, so both should be carefully assessed.

The concept of successful aging is a case in point. In this chapter, I review its history, describe its intended consequences as stated by Rowe and Kahn (1987, 1997, 1998), and consider its unintended consequences as discussed in the two previous chapters of this book and as asserted in a more critical review by Masoro (2001). I then discuss alternative concepts that have been proposed, especially the selection-optimization-compensation model of Baltes and Baltes (1990a). This chapter concludes with a proposal to treat the two models (Baltes & Baltes; Rowe & Kahn) as complementary rather than as alternative conceptualizations of successful aging, and to include the model of structural lag (Riley & Riley, 1990) as an important third element in the overall explanatory structure.

Successful Aging: The History of a Concept

Baltes and Baltes (1990b), summarizing a large body of research on functional performance in old age, chose *Successful Aging* as the title of their edited book, a term that appeared in 4 of the 12 contributed chapters. In their introductory chapter, which also presents their selection-optimization-compensation model, Baltes and Baltes point out that the concept of successful aging has appeared in the gerontological literature at least since the 1960s and that equally optimistic views about the potentialities of old age can be found in ancient writing. They cite Cicero's classic essay on old age, "Cato Major de Senectute" (trans. 1979) as a distinct example, as well as the more contemporary works of Havighurst (1963), Palmore (1979), and Williams and Wirth (1965) on the topic of aging.

These more recent authors, including Neugarten, Havighurst, and Tobin (1961), who have stressed the potentiality for activity and vigor in old age, were offering an alternative to disengagement theory (Cumming & Henry, 1961), a then influential doctrine that described the developmental task of old age as a shift from striving to withdrawing. Most gerontologists would now agree that though disengagement is an unavoidable end-of-life necessity, its theoretical proponents were urging it at an inappropriately early stage.

During the past 10 or 15 years, the concept of successful aging has become prominent in gerontological research. In 2002, the Boolean keywords "aging *and* successful" generated 246 references in the social science indices and 455 mentions in the citation indices for the biomedical and biological sciences. Scanning these references, however, reveals little agreement on either its definition or measurement. As so often happens when an ordinary phrase is appropriated for scientific purposes, "successful aging" has become an umbrella term for an assortment of more specific concepts and measures. Baltes and Baltes (1990a) cite seven outcome measures frequently used as indicators of successful aging: length of life, biological health, mental health, cognitive efficacy, social competence and productivity, personal control, and life satisfaction. Most of these, in turn, require multiple measures. They conclude that defining successful aging is in part an exercise of value judgments and one that requires "a systemic view."

In our initial article on aging, coauthor Rowe and I expressed aspirations that, though ambitious for gerontology in some respects, did not provide a precise definition of successful aging or propose specific ways of measuring it (Rowe & Kahn, 1987). The following paragraphs are excerpted from our article in *Science* in 1987:

> Research on aging has emphasized losses. In the absence of identifiable pathology, gerontologists and geriatricians have tended to interpret age-associated cognitive and physiologic deficits as age-determined. We believe that the role of aging per se in these losses has often been overstated and that a major component of many age-associated declines can be explained in terms of life style, habits, diet, and an array of psychosocial factors extrinsic to the aging process.
>
> Research on aging has also emphasized differences between age groups. The substantial heterogeneity within age groups has been either ignored or attributed to differences in genetic endowment. That perspective neglects the important impact of extrinsic factors and the interaction between psychosocial and physiologic variables. . . .
>
> Investigators . . . have from the beginning recognized the importance of separating pathologic changes from those that could be attributed to aging per se. . . . Results on the population remaining after such (physiologic) exclusions have then been interpreted as representing "normal" aging. . . .
>
> The concept of normality, explicit or implied, has served well in such research. . . . Nevertheless, the division of populations into diseased versus normal and the division of research findings into disease-related and age-determined have serious limitations. Chief among these is the neglect of heterogeneity among older people in the nondiseased group with respect to many physiologic and cognitive characteristics, a heterogeneity that is important both within cultures and between cultures. A second limitation of the emphasis on normality is the implication of harmlessness or lack of risk. And a third limitation is the related implication that what is normal is somehow natural and therefore is or should be beyond purposeful modification. In short, the emphasis on "normal" aging focuses attention on learning what most people do and do not do; what physiologic states are typical. It tends to create a gerontology of the usual. . . .

Each of the foregoing limitations urges the development of an additional conceptual distinction within the normal category, which can be approximated by the contrast between usual on the one hand and successful on the other. (pp. 143–149).

Successful Aging: A Conceptual Definition

Thus, our 1987 article (Rowe & Kahn) did not include a specific definition of successful aging, nor did it deal with questions of measurement. It was written in the early days of the MacArthur Foundation Research Network on Successful Aging, at a time when members of that interdisciplinary group had agreed on the main thrust of their collective effort but had yet to solve many of the research problems that came with it.

Ten years later, the MacArthur group had completed much of its research; Baltes and Baltes had published *Successful Aging*, and other investigators had reported work along similar lines (e.g., Abeles, Gift, & Ory, 1994; Garfein & Herzog, 1995; Hazzard, 1995), though not always with the controversial term "success" in their titles. A decade after our *Science* article on aging research, we offered a definition and conceptual framework for successful aging. The following description of successful aging is excerpted from our 1997 article in *The Gerontologist* (Rowe & Kahn):

> We define successful aging as including three main components: low probability of disease and disease-related disability, high cognitive and physical functional capacity, and active engagement with life. All three terms are relative and the relationship among them . . . is to some extent hierarchical. . . . successful aging is more than the absence of disease, important though that is, and more than the maintenance of functional capacities, important as it is. Both are important components of successful aging, but it is their combination with active engagement with life that represents the concept of successful aging most fully.

> Each of the three components of successful aging includes subparts. Low probability of disease refers not only to the absence or presence of disease itself, but also to absence, presence, or severity of risk factors for disease. High functional level includes both physical and cognitive components. [But] physical and cognitive capacities are potentials for activity; they tell us what a person *can* do, not what he or she *does* do. Successful aging goes beyond potential; it involves activity. While active

engagement with life takes many forms, we are most concerned with two—interpersonal relations and productive activity. Interpersonal relations involve contacts and transactions with others, exchange of information, emotional support, and direct assistance. An activity is productive if it creates societal value, whether or not it is reimbursed. Thus a person who cares for a disabled family member or works as a volunteer in a local church or hospital is being productive, although unpaid. (Herzog & Morgan, 1992)

Successful Aging: Critique of the Concept

Recent commentaries on successful aging, at least as we have defined them, raise a number of questions, criticisms, and proposals for improvement. The most sweeping and negative reactions to our definition appeared in a review essay by Masoro (2001). Important issues on successful aging have also been raised by Riley (1998); and by Strawbridge and Wallhagen and Rakowski, Clark, Miller, and Berg in the first two chapters of this book. I discuss the comments of all of these authors in the order in which I mentioned them.

The Masoro Review

In his 2001 review of two books on longevity, Masoro, an eminent research physiologist at the University of Texas, included a critical discussion of our 1987 *Science* article and our 1998 book *Successful Aging* (Rowe & Kahn).

Masoro's criticisms of our research on successful aging are essentially these: (a) it downplays the importance of genetics; (b) it ignores the species-determined deterioration of late life; and (c) therefore it is misleading to individuals and to policy makers. Moreover, he states that the emphasis of successful aging research on the heterogeneity of elderly populations leads to the celebration of a "fortunate elite" (successful agers) and to the neglect or blaming of those less fortunate (less successful or unsuccessful agers). Regarding Masoro's first point, he notes that our assessment of genetic contributions to successful aging is based mainly on data from the Swedish National Twin Registry, which included more than 300 pairs of twins, mean age 66 years, half of whom were reared together and half of whom were reared apart. From research on that population, we (Rowe & Kahn, 1997) had cited the following heritability coefficients—the proportion of total variance attributable to genetic factors—for major risk factors for cardiovascular and cerebrovascular disease: .66–.70 for body mass index, .28–.78 for individual lipids (total cholesterol, low- and high-density lipoprotein cholesterol, apolipoproteins A-1 and B, and triglycerides), .44 for systolic, and .34 for diastolic blood pressure (Heller, deFaire, Pedersen, Dahlen, & McClearn, 1993; Hong, deFaire, Heller, McClearn, & Pedersen, 1994; Stunkard, Harris, Pedersen, & McClearn, 1990, as cited in Rowe & Kahn, 1997).

In the same article, we indicated that "among male identical twins, the risk of death from coronary heart disease (CHD) was eightfold greater for those whose twin died before age 55" and, for female identical twins, when one died "before the age of 65, the risk of death for the other twin was 15 times greater than if one's twin did not die before the age of 65." We concluded that "intrinsic (i.e., genetic) factors alone, while highly significant, do not dominate the determination of risk in advancing age" (Rowe & Kahn, 1997, p. 435). Whether this constitutes a tendency to "downplay genetics" thus becomes a matter of judgment.

Masoro's second assertion surprised me: that we ignored the inevitable deterioration that comes in late life, typically among men and women in their 80's. My wife and I, both in our mid-80's, are keenly aware of the reduction in energy and the assorted comorbidities that are characteristic of our age range. But to turn to text rather than to anecdote, I quote from a section entitled "Successful Aging Or the Imitation of Youth?" in our 1998 book (Rowe & Kahn):

> Modern society, perhaps especially American society, seems to regard aging as something to be denied or concealed. . . [A] massive and inventive cosmetics industry does its best to persuade middle aged and elderly women—and increasingly, men—that they will lead happier lives if they change their hair color from gray to some improbable shade of blonde or red, camouflage their hair loss, and cover, erase, or abrade their wrinkles.

> Photographs that advertise the products in question show people who are invariably young in appearance; photographers and make-up artists collaborate to send the incessant message of youth. And what cosmetics and computer-enhanced photography cannot do, plastic surgery offers to accomplish. The implication of all this information and misinformation is that the ultimate form of successful aging would be no aging at all. A psychologist might be tempted to say that underlying this denial of

the aging process is a more deep-seated denial: refusal to acknowledge the fact of human mortality and the inevitability of death.

Our view of successful aging is not built on the search for immortality and the fountain of youth. . . .

In short, successful aging means just what it says—aging well, which is very different from not aging at all. The three main components of successful aging—avoiding disease and disability, maintaining mental and physical function, and continuing engagement with life—are important throughout life, but their realization in old age differs from that at earlier life stages. (pp. 48–49)

Masoro's third criticism is that the concept of successful aging celebrates a fortunate elite, which misleads individuals and leads policy makers to neglect or blame those who are less fortunate in the aging process. This is too sweeping and general a judgment to be answered by research citations or references to texts. Moreover, I assume that it was meant to apply to all who have used the term "successful aging." Rowe and I, as coauthors of publications on successful aging, intended both to encourage health-promotive behavior on the part of older men and women, and to advocate policies that facilitate and reward such behavior. The final chapter of our book, "Prescriptions for an Aging Society," describes a number of such policies.

The Riley Commentary

Issues of policy are central to Matilda Riley's (1998) commentary on our 1997 article on aging in *The Gerontologist*. She points out that the Rowe-Kahn model of successful aging "remains seriously incomplete: Although it elaborates the potentials for individual success, it fails to develop adequately the social structural opportunities necessary for realizing success" (p. 151). I find this criticism both accurate and constructive—or perhaps accurate and *challenging* come closer to the mark. Our definition of successful aging is essentially individual, and the health-promotive behaviors that improve one's chances for aging successfully must be enacted by individuals. But the factors that encourage or discourage and enable or prevent such behavior are social. Research in recent years has shown beyond question that income, education, race, neighborhood, employment status, accessibility of medical care, and many other such factors are strong predictors of life quality and even life expectancy in old age. These factors, which are expressions of societal policies and priorities, change over time, but at a pace and dynamic of their own. Changes in human lives, including life expectancy, have been occurring at a faster pace, at least for the past century. The result is a condition that Riley and her colleagues have named "structural lag"—the failure of social structures, norms, and institutions to keep pace with the metamorphosis in lives (Riley, Foner, & Waring, 1988; Riley, Huber, & Hess, 1988; Riley & Riley, 1990).

As Riley notes, our 1997 (Rowe & Kahn) article gives brief recognition to these issues in our concluding paragraph, where we say that

> many of the predictors of risk and of both functional and activity levels appear to be potentially modifiable, either by individuals or by changes in their immediate environments. The stage is thus set for intervention studies to identify effective strategies that enhance the proportion of our older population that ages successfully. (p. 149).

But I agree with Riley's conclusion that a complete model of successful aging should incorporate the external factors (environmental, institutional, societal) that enable or prevent it.

In his 1996 elaboration of the selection-optimization-compensation model, Baltes introduces the principle of "age-related increase in need (demand) for culture," and explains that "*culture* in this context refers to the entirety of psychological, social, material, and symbolic (knowledge-based) resources that humans have generated over the millennia, and which, as they are transmitted across generations, make human development possible as we know it today" (p. 368). This, it seems to me, leaves a place for the exogenous variables to which Riley refers, but it does not go further. The theoretical task that she sets has yet to be fully accomplished.

This brief critical discussion of the historical context of defining successful aging brings us to my comments on the introductory chapters of this book, which address this concept.

Strawbridge and Wallhagen: Chapter 1

The main thrust of this chapter is found in its title "Self-Rated Successful Aging: Correlates and Predictors." I consider this to be an important and constructive addition to the conceptual debate and, potentially, to the continuing flow of gerontological research. The subjective ratings by individuals of their own health are significant predictors of mortality, even when major "objective factors" are statistically controlled. In the behavioral sciences, researchers tend to rely primarily on self-reported data. Sociologists, political scientists and, to a considerable extent, economists and psychologists work with the verbal responses of individuals as their raw material.

One of the methodological lessons from this research is the importance of obtaining for major concepts both subjective (self-reported) data and, wherever possible, corresponding "objective" (independent) data. For example, stress researchers have learned that a stimulus one person reports as stressful may seem pleasantly challenging to another. If we wish to understand how people behave and what choices they make, we must understand their frames of reference.

This issue brings to mind an example from a study of quality of employment conducted many years ago (Strauss, 1972). In answer to a direct question about job satisfaction, one respondent—a factory worker with a limited educational background—stated, "I got a pretty good job." On the usual 5-point scale, that response would have been entered as "satisfied," but the interviewer also asked, "What makes it such a good job?" And to that question came an answer that indicated the worker's frame of reference:

> Don't get me wrong. I didn't say it is a *good* job. It's an OK job—about as good as a guy like me might expect. The foreman leaves me alone and it pays well. But I would never call it a *good* job. It doesn't amount to much, but it's not bad. (cited in Kahn, 1981, p. 28)

An older person might assess his or her degree of success (or health, well-being, etc.) by comparison with others of similar age; with others dealing with the same disease or disability, or with his or her own health at some earlier age or at a more recent time. In the Strawbridge-Wallhagen research, the importance of frames of reference is further illustrated by the finding that "older people rate physical functioning as no more important than other aspects of life, such as social relationships, community ties, mental health, and continued learning."

The overall assessment of the successful aging concept by Strawbridge and Wallhagen is a mix of positive and negative factors. They appreciate the shift in focus toward "those older persons who are doing well as opposed to the usual focus on the four Ds (disease, disability, dementia, and death)." They welcome the concept's encouraging "an examination of those factors that enable positive aging" and its challenge to the view that aging consists only of unrelenting declines.

On the other hand, they are concerned with difficulties of measurement—of making successful aging "operational." And they share Masoro's concern that the emphasis on successful aging "can lead to focusing on a small, elite segment of the population and thus reduce interest in secondary and tertiary prevention for the vast majority of older persons already experiencing chronic conditions and symptoms." They point out that it is "not necessarily the case that patterns observed in such an elite group will lead to useful interventions for the rest of the older population."

I have addressed the criticism of elitism earlier in response to Masoro's concerns, but Strawbridge and Wallhagen raise the additional question of whether or not studies of elite groups generate findings that are useful for more representative populations. The answer, of course, is that we do not know in all cases, and therefore researchers who aspire to generalize specific findings to broader populations must include representatives of those populations in their designs. The MacArthur community-based studies of successful aging did exactly that; their samples included the full range of the community-dwelling older adult population, not just the high performers.

Strawbridge and Wallhagen raise an additional important point: the ability of physical functioning among older people. They observe that even short-term variations between ability and disability are common. Surveys typically attempt to deal with such issues by linking their questions to specific time periods or by using language to avoid short-term, atypical events. Preambles like "Of course, everybody gets sick now and then, but on the whole would you say . . ." are common. They may avoid the unwanted intrusion of short-term changes, but they also fail to measure their effects. In one of the studies by the MacArthur group, residents of a retirement community had weekly assessments of biomedical, cognitive, and physical functioning for a period of 25 weeks (Eizenman, Nesselroade, Featherman, & Rowe, 1997; Kim, Nesselroade, & Featherman, 1996). The same measurements were taken from a matched control group at the beginning and end of the 25–week period. Within-person variability of an index based on gait, balance, and blood pressure was a strong predictor of mortality 5 years later ($R = .70$).

This and similar findings led us to call intra-individual variability "a newly identified risk factor in older persons" (Rowe & Kahn, 1997). We speculated that if we had continuous rather than occasional measures of successful aging, we would expect to find that even older people who are aging successfully have not met the criteria at every moment in the past. They have moved 'in and out of success,' just as healthy people can be said to move in and out of illness. (p. 439).

We proposed the concept of *resilience* to describe the rapidity and completeness with which people recover from episodes of stress, whether illness, accident, bereavement, or other such events. As they stand, neither the Rowe-Kahn model nor the Baltes and Baltes model deals explicitly with the issue of short-term variability, its causes and its effects.

On balance, Strawbridge and Wallhagen express a preference for the Baltes and Baltes (1990) model of selection-optimization-compensation, which they believe describes successful aging as "doing the best one can with what one has" and thus makes it a more attainable goal for the elderly population as a whole.

Rakowski et al.: Chapter 2

This chapter enlarges the discussion of successful aging in several respects: (a) It deals with a population who are not usually included in research on successful aging namely, residents in assisted living facilities; (b) it concentrates on reciprocity (giving support as well as receiving it) as a factor in successful aging," and (c) it includes the perceptions of staff members as well as residents regarding the meaning of successful aging under the special circumstances of assisted living.

All three are welcome developments in gerontological research, as is the excellent introductory section that sets successful aging in the historical context of other gerontologically optimistic concepts, namely, the "discovery" of continued mental plasticity in old age, the apparent tendency toward compression of morbidity, and the distinction between fluid and crystallized intelligence. As for successful aging, Rakowski and his coauthors conclude that

a major empirical and philosophical challenge has been to establish definitions of success that allow a broad range of older persons to be included, rather than to establish definitions that exclude groups of the population on a virtually a priori basis because they do not meet the criteria posed for optimal aging.

Their two basic premises are (a) that success should be redefined to "allow even people with multiple illnesses and functional impairments the possibility of being classified as aging successfully"; and (b) that "success at aging should *not* imply that some older persons will be automatically labeled as 'aging unsuccessfully.'" They conclude that the model of selective optimization with compensation appears to avoid these problems because "in essence, this approach defines those who are successfully aging as individuals who choose to make the best use of the capacities and resources they still have, despite illness and functional problems, while finding ways to compensate for these limitations."

I share the concerns of these authors that the Rowe-Kahn definition of successful aging, or the label itself, may have had the unintended effect of defining the majority of the elderly population as unsuccessful, that is, as failing to age successfully. However, I suspect this problem has less to do with lexicography than with contemporary American culture. We Americans seem locked into a dichotomous all-or-nothing, succeed-or-fail view of the world, in spite of the natural world's constant reminders that (with a few important exceptions like the distinction between being dead and alive) continua rather than dichotomies are the stuff of life.

In the case of success versus failure, our cultural preference for dichotomies is complicated by a benign wish that no one should fail, or at least not suffer the ego-assaulting experience of being so classified. I will resist the temptation to illustrate this point with a long digression about the unintended effect of a "nobody fails" approach in our age-graded system of public education.

It may be that the solution to this problem is to avoid entirely the language of success, with the attendant implication of failure as its obverse. Certainly Rowe and I intended to emphasize a multidimensional concept of successful aging, in which most people would find themselves doing very well on some dimensions and less well on others. As dramatic exemplars of this point, we cited Stephen Hawking, Franklin Delano Roosevelt, and Mother Teresa, all of whose lives demonstrate remarkable success in many respects, in spite of undeniable disabilities (Rowe & Kahn, 1998, p. 38). The pragmatic question remains: Are researchers, practitioners, and the relevant public enlightened and motivated, or misled and discouraged, by an approach to successful or "ideal" aging that acknowledges its multidimensionality, encourages behaviors that maximize individual attainment within its dimensions, and honors those who excel in some dimensions while being limited in others?

Rakowski and his colleagues also prepare the introduction of reciprocity as a factor in successful aging and I agree that it is important, especially if we enlarge the concept of reciprocity itself beyond the more usual limits of symmetrical and near-simultaneous exchanges in kind. I also welcome the exploration of the assisted living residents' own criteria of successful aging, invited by Rakowski and his colleagues. The mention by these older adults of being physically active, maintaining good health, and keeping in touch with friends fits easily into the three main components of the Rowe–Kahn model. But residents' emphasis on "being proud of family and children" and "keeping a positive outlook" puts these additional cognitive/perceptual/affective elements among the defining components of successful aging. I hope that Rakowski and his colleagues will pursue these findings in their subsequent work and that other gerontologists who share their interest in successful aging will reach beyond the usual community-dwelling populations.

Conclusions

Several of the coauthors of this book have suggested that the Baltes selection-optimization-compensation model and the Rowe-Kahn model of successful aging may be complementary rather than oppositional. I share this view, and I would enlarge the complementarity to include the Riley (1988) model of structural lag as the result of two interdependent but differently paced societal processes, the *dynamism of changing lives* and the *dynamism of structural change*.

The relationship among the three models can be stated in somewhat oversimplified form as follows: The Baltes model of selection, optimization, and compensation emphasizes doing the best with what you have—physically, mentally, and situationally. Accordingly, Baltes and Baltes (1990a) offer the example of the great pianist Arthur Rubinstein who explained his ability to continue concert performances in old age by limiting his repertoire (selection), practicing much more than he used to (optimization), and giving the impression of great speed when it was called for, by deliberately reducing the tempo of preceding passages (compensation).

The Rowe-Kahn model emphasizes what individuals themselves can do to improve or maintain what they have—their physical and mental capacities. For example, diet and nutrition, aerobic and resistive exercise, immunization, and early diagnosis of symptoms are in large part matters of individual choice. Activities that are mentally stimulating—reading, chess, crossword puzzles, and the like—are also options for aging adults.

Also, the Riley model emphasizes what societies can do, through law and custom, to provide the external resources that increase individuals' opportunities and thus facilitate the behaviors that make for success. Early diagnosis of symptoms, for example, is more likely when good medical facilities are easily accessed and costs are covered by insurance. Neighborhood walks for exercise are more tempting when neighborhoods are attractive and safe. Involvement in voluntary organizations, often recommended for older people, may require convenient public transportation.

Advocates for each model might point out it each includes to some extent the central points of the others. Thus, the Baltes model, especially in his 1996 elaboration, refers to the age-related increase in need (demand) for culture, and stipulates that "culture in this context refers to the entirety of psychological, social, material, and symbolic (knowledge-based) resources that humans have generated over the millennia, and which, as they are transmitted across generations, make human development possible as we know it today" (p. 378).

In the final chapter of *Successful Aging,* we state that our "emphasis has been on what people themselves can do to age successfully" (Rowe and Kahn, 1998, p. 378). Now we shift gears, thinking at the level of community facilities and national policy. Decisions and resources at community, state, and national levels affect the probability that each of us can age successfully. Finally, we consider the policy changes that might make successful aging the majority experience and imagine the contributions that a majority of successful agers could make to the larger society.

Riley and Riley (1994), having discussed the two dynamisms and the sources and consequences of their asynchrony, allow themselves to imagine an age-integrated society in which that asynchrony and the resulting mismatch between older people's capacities and society's opportunity structures have been resolved. The result, they speculate, would be "a reconstruction of people's entire lives. . . . People in their later years would find doors opening to the full range of role choices, and they could become popularly regarded as an asset, not a burden on society" (p. 29).

Thus, each of the models reaches toward the other, but each has its own emphasis. Their complete integration is a theoretical task for the future. Meanwhile, I think the concept of successful aging can serve us well, despite the discomfort it has evoked from some of our colleagues. As a concluding comment on the subject, I cite a prescient passage in the chapter by Baltes and Baltes (1990) in which they first proposed their model of selection-optimization-compensation as a way of defining success in aging. After admitting that such success might seem intellectually and emotionally paradoxical, they added:

> There is also the possible critique that the notion of successful aging may be a latent vestige of social Darwinism, a rampant competitive spirit, and one of the less desirable excesses of Western capitalist traditions. Even the last phase of life, critics can argue, is about to be captured by the view that success, defined by standards external to the individual, is a necessary part of the good life.

> At second glance, however, the association of aging with success might indicate that the apparent contradiction is intended to provoke a probing analysis of the nature of old age as it exists today. We are asked not only to reflect upon but also to participate in the creation of aging, instead of passively experiencing it as a given reality that is "natural" only for the reason that it exists. In this sense, the concept of successful aging suggests a vigorous examination of what might in principle be possible. Moreover, a critical but constructive analysis of the concept may indeed serve to articulate the idea that forms and vehicles of "success" in old age may be different from those in earlier phases of life. (Baltes & Baltes, 1990, p. 4)

I can imagine no more eloquent defense of the concept of successful aging. The chapters in this book have met for me the Baltes's criteria of critical but constructive analysis, and I hope that they will do as much for other readers.

Chapter 4

Health Expectancy: An Indicator of Successful Aging and a Measure of the Impact of Chronic Disease and Disability

Eileen M. Crimmins, Jung Ki Kim, and Aaron Hagedorn

W hen the 20th century began, death from infectious disease was common. People who died of infectious diseases were often ill for only a short time before death. Life expectancy was approximately 40 years and many people did not survive childhood. Under these conditions, life expectancy was a good indicator of the health of the population. At the beginning of the 21st century, things are quite different. Life expectancy has almost doubled to 75 years, and most people die in old age of a chronic condition that has developed and from which they have often suffered for a number of years. When death is primarily caused by chronic conditions that are concentrated at the older ages, health expectancy is a useful indicator of the average length of time a person will live with good health.

Health expectancy, or the expected length of life without disease and disability, can be used to clarify the relative length of time the population lives free of different health conditions. Thus, the difference between total life expectancy and healthy life expectancy is the length of life lived with a health problem. These numbers can be the basis of policy making in that estimates of life spent with certain diseases and disabilities can be linked to estimates of the potential for treating or eliminating these diseases as well as associated costs to help make resource allocation decisions. These estimates also serve as useful indicators of differentials in the burden of health problems that arise from different diseases and conditions.

Background

Until recently, health trends and differences have been primarily indicated by mortality levels. Life expectancy is often used as a summary measure of an extensive set of age-specific mortality rates. Because life expectancy is not affected by population age-structure, values can be compared for different social, demographic, or national groups at one point or for the same groups over time. In addition, because life expectancy is expressed in years, its meaning is easily understood by both policy makers and the public.

The desire to develop comparable composite measures that divide life into healthy and unhealthy years has derived from the recent interest in monitoring change in quality as well as quantity of life (Olshansky & Wilkins, 1998). As later life has become a time when most people live with one or more chronic conditions, there is an interest in improving not just the quantity but also the quality of life (U.S. Department of Health and Human Services [USDHHS], 1998). The U.S. government now has stated goals in terms of increasing the length of quality of life as well as the total quantity of life (USDHHS). Therefore, measures of health expectancy provide a useful basis for assessing progress toward such a goal, which has resulted in their use by international groups such as the World Health Organization and the World Bank (Murray & Lopez, 1997) and the European Union (Robine, 2000). In addition, many individual countries have adopted such measures, including the United States (Erickson, Wilson & Shannon, 1995; Molla, Wagener, & Mordans, 2001).

The health expectancy approach can be used to indicate the average length of time spent with any dimension of morbidity or poor health: diseases, conditions or impairments, and functioning losses or disability. These are all distinct dimensions of what has been termed the disability process (Verbrugge & Jette, 1994). In surveyed populations, the loss of ability usually begins with the onset of diseases and conditions of older age, proceeds to functioning loss and eventual disability, and ends in death. Although measures linking dimensions of health and mortality were proposed more than 30 years ago (Sanders, 1964; Sullivan, 1971), it is only in the last 10 years that substantial work has been done to develop summary measures to estimate the years lived without various diseases and disabilities (Murray, Salomen, & Mathers, 1999; Saito, Crimmins, & Hayward, 1999). Such measures are informative for indicating the relative burden of different diseases and conditions for the population as a whole and for different demographic groups in the population. For instance, it is useful to clarify whether longer-lived groups such as women and White people also experience shorter years with disability and disease and longer years in good health.

In this chapter, we estimate the number of years lived with and without a variety of health conditions for the U.S. community-dwelling population in 1994. In addition, we examine the differential burden of disease and disability for men and women, Blacks and other populations, and at birth and at age 65. It is very clear from our estimates that most of the disease and disability that burden the population occurs in the older ages.

Data

The measures estimated in this chapter have been developed using age-specific mortality rates by sex and sometimes by race from 1994 national vital statistics data. These rates are adjusted for subsequent changes in estimates of the population size and are available on the Web site of the National Center for Health Statistics (2001).

Age-specific estimates of the prevalence of health problems are derived from the annual National Health Interview Survey of the United States. This survey is an annual ongoing national sample of approximately 50,000 households and 100,000 individuals representative of the resident civilian population (Adams & Marrano, 1995). These estimates of unhealthy life do not include the institutionalized population. Estimates of the prevalence of disability and self-reported health are from the 1994 survey. That year, 116,179 people were interviewed; of these, 14,571 were 65 or over. Most respondents were White (89,571), but data were collected from a substantial number of Blacks (16,462) and others (5,135). Three years of survey data, from 1993, 1994, and

1995, are used to estimate the length of life with disease. This is because the annual sample is divided into six subsamples in the section addressing disease prevalence, and data for 1 year do not produce reliable estimates.

All National Health Interview Survey respondents indicate long-term disability through responses to questions about their ability to perform activities related to their usual social role. In this survey, which is designed to monitor the health and disability of the U.S. population, long-term disability is defined as limitation in activity. Depending on age and behavior, usual activity can include playing, attending school, working or keeping house, or living independently. People who report themselves as unable to perform or limited in their normal social role are classified as having some disability. People then are asked about other activities, including leisure and social activities; persons limited in their ability to do these activities are also classified as having a disability.

More severe disability is measured in the population through responses to questions on their ability to perform personal care and perform tasks necessary for independent living. These questions, which are analogous to those typically used to measure the presence of difficulty in performing activities of daily living (ADL) or instrumental activities of daily living (IADL), take the following form: "Because of any impairment or health problem, do you need the help of other persons with personal care needs, such as eating, bathing, dressing, or getting around this home?" and "Because of any impairment or health problem, do you need the help of other persons in handling routine needs, such as household chores, doing necessary business, shopping, or getting around for other purposes?" A positive answer to the first question indicates a person unable to provide all of his or her own care, and a positive response to the second indicates someone who needs help with independent living. Children younger than age 17 are all assumed to need help with these activities, but they are not classified as disabled.

A comprehensive personal assessment of health status is provided by people's answers to the following question: "Would you say your health in general is excellent, very good, good, fair, or poor?" We examine the length of life in good health defined by answering *good, very good,* or *excellent* health. Life not in good health is defined by an answer of *fair* or *poor* health.

Life without disease is based on estimates of the prevalence of major chronic conditions. People are asked if they have ever had heart disease, hypertension, arthritis, asthma, or chronic bronchitis or emphysema. They are also asked if in the past 12 months they have had diabetes (Adams & Marano, 1995).

Methods

To determine the years of life with and without disability and with and without disease, we use the cross-sectional approach to healthy life expectancy described by Crimmins, Saito, and Ingegneri (1989; 1997). The basis of this approach is to divide the life-table value for years lived in an age interval $_5L_x$ into years lived with and without a health condition by multiplying the life table $_5L_x$ value by the proportion of the persons in the age group with the health condition. Doing this for each age group produces two L_x columns, which are then summed for each age and higher to provide two T_x columns or years lived with and without disease at each age. These values are divided by the number of persons entering each age group to provide estimates of the expectation of life e_x, with and without the health condition of interest at each age.

These measures can be computed for all ages; in Crimmins et al. (1989, 1997), they are shown at birth, and at ages 30 and 65. Significantly, even when the measure is computed at birth, the health of those above age 65 years is the most important influence on the estimate of the total number of years lived over a lifetime with a health problem for most aspects of health examined. This is a characteristic of all life-table-based estimates where most morbidity and mortality occur at the oldest ages.

There have been a number of different approaches to estimating healthy life that seemingly provide comparable indicators; however, some approaches are based on quite different assumptions. They differ from the measure used here in that they combine multiple attributes of health and/or they weight the health states according to the severity of the health problem or both. For instance, the U.S. government has used a measure called Years of Healthy Life in setting goals for the years 2000 and 2010. This measure is based on a composite of self-reported health and disability indicators. The composite health states in this measure are then weighted to estimate years of healthy life, which represent years lived in perfect health after the value of years lived in less than perfect health has been subtracted. Weights range from 1.0 for a person in excellent health with no disability to 0.0, which is death. Disabled and unhealthy states are in between. The average weight for life lived after age 85 in the official calculations is about .5 (Erickson et al., 1995). This results in an estimate of total years lived that does not reflect either average years lived healthy or unhealthy but rather weighted years. A weighting approach is also used in the Adjusted Health Expectancies produced by the World Health Organization in the Global Burden of Disease Project (Murray & Lopez, 1997).

We do not weight years of life in the approach used in this chapter because we feel is that weighting produces information that is less informative, particularly for the older population. Estimates of life lived that are reported in this chapter are of years lived with and without a series of health problems.

Results

Estimates of the length of healthy and unhealthy life according to a number of indicators are shown in Tables 4.1 and 4.2. Table 4.1 shows figures at birth; Table 4.2 contains indicators for age 65. Both tables contain figures for the total population as well as for men and women.

Life expectancy at birth was 75.7 in 1994; 62 of these years were lived without any disability, and all but 14 of the years were lived able

Table 4.1 Healthy and Unhealthy Life Expectancy at Birth

	Total population	Males	Females	Difference females–males
Expected Years of Life at Birth—Total	75.7	72.6	78.8	6.2
Free of any disability	62.1	60.3	64.0	3.7
Able to perform personal care and routine needs	71.9	70.2	73.8	3.6
Able to perform personal care	74.3	71.5	77.1	5.6
In good health or better	66.4	64.4	68.4	4.0
With any disability	13.6	12.3	14.8	2.5
Unable to perform personal care or routine needs	3.8	2.4	5.0	2.6
Unable to perform personal care	1.4	1.1	1.7	0.6
Not in good health or better	9.3	8.2	10.4	2.2

Note: Based on 1994 mortality and health information from the 1994 NHIS.

Table 4.2 Healthy and Unhealthy Life Expectancy at Age 65

	Total population	Males	Females	Difference females–males
Expected Years of Life at Age 65—Total	17.4	15.8	18.8	3.0
Free of any disability	10.5	9.8	11.1	1.3
Able to perform personal care and routine needs	14.3	14.0	14.8	0.8
Able to perform personal care	16.2	14.8	17.2	2.4
In good health or better	12.5	11.2	13.5	2.3
With any disability	6.9	6.0	7.7	1.7
Unable to perform personal care or routine needs	3.1	1.8	4.0	2.2
Unable to perform personal care	1.2	1.0	1.6	0.6
Not in good health or better	4.9	4.6	5.3	0.7

Note: Based on 1994 mortality and health information from the 1994 NHIS.

to perform personal care. At age 65, people can expect to live 17.4 years, of which 10.5 will be free of any disability. At age 65, the average person who is not currently institutionalized can expect to spend about a year needing some help or having some difficulty performing personal care and almost 3 years having some difficulty with the tasks needed for independent living. A comparison of Tables 4.1 and 4.2 indicates that most of the years of severe disability and about half of all disabled years are lived over the age of 65.

Life expectancy for women is 78.8 years—longer than the 72.6 years for men. Women will be free of any disability for 64 of those years and able to live independently and take care of themselves for almost 74 years. On average, women live 77 years able to perform all ADLs. This means that women spend about 15 years with some disability. Most of these years are with moderate disability; about 5 years of help with personal care and routine needs are required. Men live fewer years and fewer disabled years, using any of these definitions of disability. They live 12 years with some disability and only 1 year needing help with personal care. The largest differential between men and women is in the length of time during which they cannot live independently (i.e., need help with routine needs or personal care). Though women live 5 years in this state, men only live half as long.

Note that the numbers for age 65 imply very different average ages of disability onset than those for age 0 or birth. Among people who are age 65, the expected length of life without any disability is 10 years for men and 11 years for women. This means that a man of age 65 can expect to live to 75 without even moderate disability, and a woman can expect to live to 76 with moderate disability. Women at age 65 can expect to live longer than men in each healthy state and each unhealthy state (Table 4.2).

Self-Assessed Health

Self-assessed health can be regarded as a personal evaluation of a health state, taking into account all available information about the disease, all problems related to disability and functioning loss, and some reference for evaluating appropriate health. Both men and women spend most of their lives, from birth or from age 65, reporting that their health is at least *good* (Tables 4.1 and 4.2). Only about 5 years after age 65 are spent with health that is assessed as at least *good,* which is fairly similar for men and women. The average age at which health is assessed as less than good is older than the average age at onset of any disability. This means that on average, people with some disabilities still assess their health as *good* or *better.*

Life With and Without Disease

We also estimate years lived with specific diseases and conditions, which we regard as the beginning of the disability process. Years lived with and without a set of diseases—heart disease, arthritis, diabetes, hypertension, asthma, bronchitis or emphysema—for the entire life span and after age 65 are shown in Tables 4.3 and 4.4. The diseases with which people spend the most years are arthritis and hypertension. On average, a person spends 12 years with arthritis and 11 years with hypertension over a lifetime. Most of these years are lived after age 65, namely, 8 for arthritis and 6 for hypertension. Almost half of life after age 65 (47%) is lived with arthritis, and about a third (37%) with hypertension. These are both major problems for older age as arthritis is a primary cause of disability, and hypertension is a major cardiovascular risk factor.

Men and women have a similar length of life with heart disease, but women live significantly longer with arthritis and hypertension (Table 4.3). Women become hypertensive 3 years later than men on average

Table 4.3 Life Expectancy with and Without Diseases/Conditions at Birth by Sex (NHIS 93–95)

	Total		Males		Females	
	Years	Percentage of LE	Years	Percentage of LE	Years	Percentage of LE
Expected Years at Birth—						
Total	75.7	100.0	72.6	100.0	78.8	100.0
Without heart disease	69.0	91.1	66.3	91.3	72.0	91.4
Without arthritis	63.5	83.9	63.8	87.9	63.6	80.7
Without diabetes	72.5	95.8	69.9	96.3	75.4	95.7
Without hypertension	64.8	85.6	63.4	87.3	66.6	84.5
Without asthma	71.5	94.5	69.4	95.6	74.0	93.9
Without bronchitis/ emphysema	70.7	93.4	68.6	94.5	73.1	92.8
With heart disease	6.7	8.9	6.3	8.7	6.8	8.6
With arthritis	12.2	16.1	8.8	12.1	15.2	19.3
With diabetes	3.2	4.2	2.7	3.7	3.4	4.3
With hypertension	10.9	14.4	9.2	12.7	12.2	15.5
With asthma	4.2	5.5	3.2	4.4	4.8	6.1
With bronchitis/ emphysema	5.0	6.6	4.0	5.5	5.7	7.2

Note: Based on mortality and health information from the 1993–1995 NHIS.

(66.6 years), but they both get arthritis at about the same average age (64 years). Some of women's longer life with disease is related to their longer survival with the disease rather than an earlier age of onset. For instance, the average woman lives longer with heart disease than the average man even though her average age at onset is about 6 years later.

Race Differences in the Length of Healthy Life

We can compare the length of life in health states for Blacks, Whites, and others, using measures of healthy life expectancy (Tables 4.5, 4.6, 4.7). The longest life expectancy in the U.S. is for persons in "other" race groups—primarily Asians. This group has a life expectancy that exceeds that of Whites by about 4 years for men and 3 years for

Table 4.4 Life Expectancy with and Without Diseases/Conditions at Age 65 by Gender

	Total		Males		Females	
	Years	Percentage of LE	Years	Percentage of LE	Years	Percentage of LE
Expected Years at 65—						
Total	17.4	100.0	15.8	100.0	18.8	100.0
Without heart disease	13.1	75.3	11.4	72.2	14.5	77.1
Without arthritis	9.3	53.4	9.6	60.8	8.9	47.3
Without diabetes	15.5	89.1	14.1	89.2	16.7	88.8
Without hypertension	11.0	63.2	10.7	67.7	11.2	59.6
Without asthma	16.7	96.0	15.2	96.2	17.9	95.2
Without bronchitis/ emphysema	15.9	91.4	14.3	90.5	17.3	92.0
With heart disease	4.3	24.7	4.4	27.8	4.3	22.9
With arthritis	8.1	46.6	6.2	39.2	9.9	52.7
With diabetes	1.9	10.9	1.7	10.8	2.1	11.2
With hypertension	6.4	36.8	5.1	32.3	7.6	40.4
With asthma	0.7	4.0	0.6	3.8	0.9	4.8
With bronchitis/ emphysema	1.5	8.6	1.5	9.5	1.5	8.0

Note: Based on mortality and health information from the 1993–1995 NHIS.

Table 4.5 Healthy and Unhealthy Life Expectancy at Birth by Race

	Males			Females		
	White	Black	Others	White	Black	Others
Life Expectancy at Birth Total	73.5	65.1	77.6	79.4	73.8	82.2
Free of any disability	61.3	52.4	67.0	64.8	57.4	67.9
Able to perform personal care	72.4	64.0	76.6	77.8	71.6	80.1
Able to perform personal care and routine needs	71.0	61.9	75.5	74.6	67.7	76.4
In good health or better	65.8	54.3	67.3	69.9	58.1	68.3
With any disability	12.2	12.7	10.6	14.6	16.4	14.3
Unable to perform personal care	1.1	1.1	1.0	1.6	2.2	2.1
Unable to perform personal care or routine needs	2.5	3.2	2.1	4.8	6.1	5.8
Not in good health or better	7.7	10.8	10.3	9.5	15.7	13.9

Note: Based on 1994 mortality and health information from the 1994 NHIS.

Table 4.6 Healthy and Unhealthy Life Expectancy at Age 65 by Race

	Males			Females		
	White	Black	Others	White	Black	Others
Life Expectancy—Total	15.9	13.9	18.4	18.9	17.2	20.8
Free of any disability	10.0	7.8	13.1	11.3	8.7	12.6
Able to perform personal care	15.0	12.9	17.6	17.4	15.1	19.0
Able to perform personal care and routine needs	13.9	11.1	17.0	15.1	12.3	15.9
In good health or better	11.5	7.6	10.9	12.0	7.5	12.0
With any disability	5.9	6.1	5.3	7.6	8.5	8.2
Unable to perform personal care	0.9	1.0	0.8	1.5	2.1	1.8
Unable to perform personal care or routine needs	2.0	2.8	1.4	3.8	4.9	4.9
Not in good health or better	4.4	6.3	7.5	6.9	9.7	8.8

Note: Based on 1994 mortality and health information from the 1994 NHIS.

women (Table 4.5). Life expectancy for Whites exceeds that of Blacks by about 8 years for men and 6 years for women.

In general, Whites have longer healthy lives than Blacks, and those in the "other" category have the longest healthy lives as well as the longest lives (Table 4.5). Blacks generally spend more years with disability even though they do not live as long as other groups, although there are some exceptions to this generalization. For example, men of all races live about 1 year unable to perform personal care. Men in the "other" racial category tend to be less disabled than Whites or Blacks. This is not true for "other" women. The "other" group tends to have a level of disability that is higher and self-assessed health that is worse than might be expected on the basis of their mortality. After age 65, most of the same generalizations can be drawn (Table 4.6).

Whites of both genders live longer than Blacks after age 30, without each of the diseases examined; this is also true for the most part at age 65 (Table 4.7). These longer healthy years for Whites are an important indicator of the more successful aging of people of higher socio-economic status. Whites spend more years with some diseases (heart disease and asthma), and Blacks live more years with others (diabetes, hypertension). These differences indicate the potential for a longer life to be related to more time with diseases and less time with others.

Table 4.7 Life Expectancy at ages 30 and 65 with Diseases and Conditions, and Longer Years Lived by Whites without Diseases at Age 30 and Age 65 (1993–1995 NHIS)

	Difference in years without conditions		Years with conditions			
	Males	Females	Males		Females	
	(White–Black)	(White–Black)	White	Black	White	Black
Expected years at 30	6.7	4.5	45.4	38.7	50.5	46.0
Heart disease	3.8	3.7	6.4	3.5	6.2	5.4
Arthritis	5.3	4.8	9.0	7.6	15.1	15.4
Diabetes	7.7	7.3	2.7	3.7	2.9	5.7
Hypertension	7.0	9.1	9.1	9.4	11.4	16.0
Asthma	6.4	4.4	1.6	1.3	2.9	2.8
Bronchitis/ emphysema	5.2	3.7	2.9	1.4	4.2	3.4
Expected years at 65	2.0	1.7	15.9	13.9	18.9	17.2
Heart disease	−0.4	0.9	4.7	2.3	4.3	3.5
Arthritis	2.0	2.7	6.2	6.2	9.8	10.8
Diabetes	2.7	3.3	1.6	2.3	1.9	3.5
Hypertension	2.7	2.7	5.0	5.7	7.5	8.5
Asthma	1.9	1.7	0.6	0.5	0.9	0.9
Bronchitis/ emphysema	1.3	1.6	1.6	0.9	1.5	1.4

Note: Based on 1994 mortality and health information from the 1993–1995 NHIS.

Chapter Seven Tables

Conclusions

Healthy life expectancy provides a useful indicator of how mortality and morbidity combine to produce an average length of healthy life for the population. The difference between healthy life expectancy and total life expectancy provides a measure of the burden of diseases and disability in the population. These indicators provide a picture of the differential burden of ill health for population subgroups.

Most severe disability and life with chronic disease is lived after the age of 65. Comparison of gender differences in life without disability and total life expectancy indicates that there is less difference between men and women in the length of healthy life than in total life. This fact arises because women have a longer life with disability even though they have lower mortality. An examination of race differences shows that differences in length of disabled lives for Blacks and Whites are even greater than the differences in total life expectancy. This fact arises from the higher levels of both mortality and disability experienced by the African American population.

Estimates of the length of life with disease can be used in evaluating the potential cost and value of policy, programmatic, and medical changes. For instance, an average older American with arthritis lives 8 years after age 65. The average cost of providing new drugs to the population can be estimated using this figure. Similarly, the fact that the average length of life with hypertension is 6 years can be used to evaluate the impact of health promotion activities to delay the onset of hypertension and related heart disease.

Chapter 5

Risk and Protective Factors for Physical Functioning in Older Adults With and Without Chronic Conditions: The MacArthur Study of Successful Aging[1]

Teresa Seeman and Xinguang Chen

Older age continues to be seen largely as a period of declining health and functioning. However, the past decade has seen a renewed attention to the fact that such declines may not be inevitable and are certainly not experienced uniformly by all older adults (Butler & Gleason, 1985; Rowe & Kahn, 1987, 1998). As a growing body of research attests, risks for declines in health and functioning at older ages are influenced by lifestyle characteristics, including differences in levels of physical activity as well as levels of social engagement and psychological characteristics (Albert et al., 1995; Seeman et al., 1995; see also Seeman, 1994 for review).

Identification of factors that influence risks for functional disability is of growing importance in light of current population trends which

[1]From "Risk and Protective Factors for Physical Functioning in Older Adults with and Without Chronic Conditions: MacArthur Studies of Successful Aging" by Teresa Seeman and Xinguang Chen, 2002, *Journals of Gerontology* Swiss B, Psychological Sciences and Social Sciences, 57, S135–S144. Copyright 2002 by The Gerontological Society of America. Reproduced with permission of the Gerontological Society of America in the formal textbook via copyright Clearance Center, Inc.

project a population of some 39 million adults aged 65 and older in the next 15 years and more than 80 million of this population by 2050 (U.S. Bureau of the Census, 1996). Because risks for functional disabilities rise with age, there is considerable debate about whether this growing population of older adults will be characterized by a compression of morbidity (i.e., with disease and disability postponed to later ages) or whether people will simply live longer with greater burdens of disease and disability (Fries & Crapo, 1981; Guralnik & Schneider, 1987).

One area of interest relates to the question of whether the presence of major chronic health conditions such as diabetes, hypertension, heart disease, cancer, or broken bones is necessarily associated with declines in functioning. This is of particular significance at older ages because the risks for such chronic conditions increase significantly with advancing age so that older adults are at relatively higher risk of experiencing one or more such conditions. The majority of research on models of physical functioning at older ages has focused on analyses of the older population as a whole, adjusting for differences in health status (i.e., the presence of various health conditions) when examining the impact of other lifestyle and demographic factors. Studies that have directly compared levels of functioning for those with and without chronic conditions have shown that chronic medical conditions have a negative association with levels of physical functioning (Stewart et al., 1989; Verbrugge & Patrick, 1995). Studies have also documented differences in lifestyle and psychosocial characteristics such as exercise, smoking, depression and self-efficacy across groups characterized by differences in health status (Ormel et al., 1997; Pennihx et al., 1998). However, with the exception of a few studies of rheumatoid arthritis (RA), there has been little attention to the potential influence of individual differences in such factors on within-group variations in levels of functioning for those with chronic conditions.

Studies of RA have shown that social and psychological factors predict differences in functional disability—being married, having a larger social network and receiving more emotional support have each been found to predict better levels of functioning (Verbrugge, Gates, & Ike, 1991) and less decline in functioning (Brown, Wallston, & Nicassio, 1989; Evers, Kraaimaat, Geenen, & Bijlsma, 1998; Leigh & Fries, 1992; Ward & Leigh, 1993). In RA and in chronic obstructive pulmonary disease, beliefs about the controllability of the disease have also been found to predict better functioning (Narsavage, 1997; Scharloo et al., 1998). A small literature also suggests that social integration and/or social support protect against functional declines post-stroke (Colantonio, Kasl, Ostfeld, & Berkman, 1993; Glass & Maddox, 1992).

In this article, we explore the general hypothesis that lifestyle and psychosocial factors that have been shown to influence risks for functional decline in the general population of older adults are consequential for population subgroups with chronic conditions. Factors hypothesized to protect against functional declines include higher socioeconomic status (i.e., more education and/or income), participation in regular physical activity, greater social engagement with others, and more positive psychological characteristics such as stronger self-efficacy beliefs and fewer symptoms of psychological distress. Using data for a 2.5 year follow-up, we test the hypothesis that such lifestyle, demographic, and psychosocial factors influence risks for declines in physical functioning over time within groups of older adults with hypertension, diabetes, cardiovascular disease, cancer, and broken bones. We also examine the impact of such factors on changes in functioning within a subgroup of adults reporting no chronic conditions.

Methods

Data for these analyses come from the MacArthur Foundation Research Network on Successful Aging, a longitudinal study of relatively high functioning men and women aged 70 to 79. As described in greater detail elsewhere (Berkman et al., 1993), subjects were subsampled on the basis of age and physical and cognitive functioning from three community-based cohorts—in Durham, North Carolina; East Boston, Massachusetts, and New Haven, Connecticut—that were part of the NIA's Established Populations for the Epidemiological Study of the Elderly (Cornoni-Huntley, Brock, Ostfeld, Taylor, & Wallace, 1986). Age-eligible 70–79 years men and women ($N = 4,030$) were screened on the basis of four criteria of physical functioning and two criteria of cognitive functioning to identify those functioning in the top third of the age group. The selection criteria included (a) no reported disability on the seven–item Activities of Daily Living (ADL) scale (Katz, Ford, Moskowitz, Jackson, & Jaffe, 1963); (b) no more than one reported mild disability on eight items tapping gross mobility and range of motion (Nagi, 1976; Rosow & Breslau, 1966); (c) ability to hold a semitandem balance for at least 10 seconds; (d) ability to stand from a seated position five times within 20 seconds; (e) scores of 6 or more correct on the nine–item SPMSQ (Short Portable Mental Status Questionnaire) Pfeiffer, 1975); and f) ability to remember three or more of six elements on a delayed recall of a short story.

Of the 4,030 age-eligible men and women, a cohort of 1,313 subjects met all screening criteria; 1,189 (90.6%) agreed to participate and provided informed consent. Baseline data collection was completed between May 1988 and December 1989 and included a 90-minute, face-to-face interview covering detailed assessments of physical and cognitive functioning, health status, and social and psychological characteristics as well as other lifestyle characteristics.

The cohort was interviewed again in 1991–1992, with reassessments of all measures included in the baseline interview. A majority of the cohort were interviewed between 24 and 32 months after their baseline interview ($\bar{x}$ = 28 months). Attrition was minimal: There were 1,066 (90%) completed interviews, 59 (5%) partial or proxy interviews, 47 (4%) refusals at follow-up, and 71 (6%) deaths.

Prevalence of Chronic Conditions

Self-report data on the prevalence of five major chronic conditions were examined hypertension (HBP]) diabetes, cardiovascular disease (CVD, i.e., heart attack or stroke), cancer, and fractures. These were the conditions with sufficient numbers of prevalent cases to permit within-group analysis of factors associated with patterns of change in physical functioning (HBP N = 563; diabetes N = 155; CVD N = 154; cancer, N = 213; fractures, N = 291). Selection of these conditions for analysis was also based on available evidence indicating that self-reports for these conditions are generally accurate (e.g., percentage agreement of .86 or higher and kappas of .70 or higher as compared with medical records) Bush, Miller, Golden, & Hale, 1989; Walker, Whincup, Shaper, Lennon, & Thomson, 1998). Subjects were classified as having the condition in question if they responded affirmatively to the question of whether a doctor had ever told them that they had it. Subjects reporting more than one condition (e.g., diabetes *and* CVD) were classified into each of the disease groups for which they indicated an affirmative response so that each disease group reflects all subjects who reported that condition. Analyses examined all those reporting a given condition (i.e., whether or not they also report other comorbid conditions), with adjustments for comorbidity, as small numbers of cases precluded analyses stratified by number of comorbid conditions or presence of a single condition. Those with no reported chronic conditions (N=310) were also examined as a group.

Physical Functioning

A summary measure of physical functioning, based on five separate tests of physical ability, was used as the primary outcome. Details regarding creation of this summary scale are available elsewhere (Seeman, Charpentier et al., 1994). The five abilities assessed included timed measures of balance, gait, chair stands, foot taps, and manual ability. Two-month test-retest data for these protocols indicate that they have generally good reliability, ranging from .61 (balance) to .91 (signature). A summary measure of physical functioning ability was developed by summing scores for the five subscales. Because the ranges for the timed scores varied among the five subscales, scores for each of the subscales were rescaled to a range of 0–1 before summing them; rescaling for the five subscales was accomplished by dividing the individual's raw score by the maximum value from the 1988 (baseline) distribution. For all tests except balance, higher timed scores indicated worse performance; for these tests, the results of the division were also subtracted from 1 to reverse the order of scores so that higher scores would reflect better performance. The rescaled scores thus range from zero (*worst*) to 1 (*best*) and represent the proportion of the best possible score that the individual achieved. This summary score had a 2–month test-retest reliability of .80. The 1991 (follow-up) timed scores were also rescaled using the 1988 denominators to permit meaningful evaluation of change over time (i.e., to ensure that changes in rescaled scores on a test reflected actual change in the timed score— numerator of rescaled score—rather than a change in the denominator of the rescaled score). Summary measures of functioning in 1988 and 1991 were created by adding the rescaled subscale scores for the respective years (range each year = 0–5). Although there is no gold standard against which to validate this measure, evidence for its construct validity is provided by its significant correlation with self-reported functional status and its apparent sensitivity to changes in health status (e.g., increased morbidity and hospitalization have been shown to predict declines in functioning scores) Seeman, Charpentier, et al., 1994). Change in functioning from 1988 to 1991 is measured as the difference (1991 score less the 1988 score) so that negative scores reflect declines in functioning from baseline to follow-up.

Sociodemographic Characteristics

Information was available regarding gender, ethnicity, age, education, and income. Ethnicity was coded *White* vs. *African American*. Education was measured initially as the number years of schooling completed. For the analyses presented here, educational attainment was classified as *less than high school* versus *high school or higher* as this categorization has been shown to have the strongest relationship to physical functioning and change in functioning (Seeman et al., 1995). Based on these earlier analyses, annual household income (originally measured in $10,000 increments to $30,000+) was classified as < $10,000 versus $10,000 or more. A second dummy indicator variable was also included for *missing income data* so as to retain these latter individuals in the analyses.

Behavioral Factors

Levels of physical activity were assessed based on self-reported frequency of current leisure- and work-related activities. Each activity mentioned was classified as light, moderate, or strenuous based on intensity codes (kcal/min) adapted from Paffenbarger, Hyde, Wing, and Hsieh (1986) and Taylor et al. (1978). Summary scales were derived by multiplying the frequency of activity (five categories, ranging from *never* to *3+ times per week*) by the intensity code and summing overall activities within a given category of intensity. For the results reported here, measures of the amount of moderate and strenuous activity were examined individually and as in combination (i.e., doing moderate and/or strenuous activity). In addition to the continuous measures of amount of activity, dichotomous variables were created to allow for assessment of more specific effects of *any activity* versus *no such activity*. We report results for the continuous measure of *amount of strenuous activity* and for the dichotomous indicator of *any* versus *no moderate or strenuous activity* as these were the only two measures found to relate significantly to measured physical functioning. Cigarette smoking was assessed by self-report and subjects were classified as current, former, or never smokers as of their 1988 baseline interview. For past and current smokers, pack-years of smoking were calculated. Alcohol consumption was assessed in terms of the monthly frequency and quantity of beer, wine, and hard liquor consumption. A summary measure of ethyl alcohol consumption was created based on the quantity and frequency of each type of alcohol consumed (Armor, Polich, & Stambul, 1975).

Social Network Characteristics

Details regarding the various scales developed from the MacArthur Battery assessments of network characteristics have been reported elsewhere (Seeman, Berkman, Blazer, & Rowe, 1994). Briefly, four major indices were developed:

1. a summary measure of *social network ties,* representing the total number of children, close friends, and relatives reported by the respondent (presence or absence of a spouse was measured separately);

2. a measure of *emotional support,* reflecting how often—range = 0 *never* to 3 *frequently*—members of the respondent's social network made the respondent "feel loved and cared for" and how often they "listen when you needed to talk about worries or a problem" (scale score based on average of responses to six items reflecting spousal support (two items), support from children (two items), and support from close friends/relatives (two items);

3. a summary measure of *instrumental support* was based on the average reported frequency—range = 0 *never* to 3 *frequently*—with which network members "helped with daily tasks" and "provided information about medical, financial or family problems" (scale score is based on average of responses to six items reflecting reported spousal assistance (two items), assistance from children (two items) and assistance from close friends/relatives (two items); and

4. a summary measure of more negative aspects of social relationships.

The latter measure reflects subjects' reports as to the frequency with which their spouse, children, friends, and relatives "made too many demands on you" or "were critical of what you do." A summary measure of *demands/criticism* was constructed based on the average reported frequency of such interactions across network ties (average of 6 items; range = 0 *never* to 3 *frequently*).

Psychological Characteristics

Self-efficacy beliefs were measured based on subjects' perceptions of their own self-efficacy in nine separate life domains found to be of particular relevance to older adults (Rodin & McAvay, 1992). In addition to a summary scale, two subscales were examined: One reflects interpersonal efficacy beliefs regarding one's ability to deal with interpersonal relationships with spouse, children and relatives and friends, while the second reflects instrumental efficacy beliefs about one's perceived ability to deal with instrumental tasks relating to finances, transportation, one's living situation, and one's sense of being productive (see Seeman, Rodin, & Albert, 1993, for additional details of scaling). Personal mastery beliefs were measured using a scale developed by Pearlin and Schooler (1978). Psychological symptomatology was measured by a 50–item version of the Hopkins Symptom Checklist

(Derogatis, Lipman, Rickels, Uhlenhuth, & Covi, 1974); a subscale measuring depressive symptoms was also examined separately.

Health Status Measures

In addition to the information on the prevalent chronic conditions used to classify subjects into analysis groups, data were available on measured blood pressure, pulmonary function, relative weight, and cognitive function, as well as medication use. Pulmonary function (peak expiratory flow rate) was assessed using a mini-Wright meter (Cook et al., 1991). Relative weight was examined in terms of body mass index (BMI; kg/m^2) from self-reported height and weight, as well as waist-hip ratio (WHR), based on measured waist circumference (at the umbilicus) and hip circumference (maximal buttocks) (Lohman, Roche, & Martorell, 1988). Blood pressure was assessed according to the HDFP protocol, using the average of the second and third of three seated readings (HDFP, 1978); presence of high systolic was defined as SBP $\geq$ 140 mmHg, high diastolic as DBP $\geq$ 90 mmHg. Cognitive functioning was measured by summing scores on tests measuring memory, abstraction, spatial recognition, and spatial (copying) ability (Inouye, Albert, Mohs, Sun, & Berkman, 1993). Information on medication use was also available based on self-reports and interviewer observation of pill bottles; a single indicator of any medication use (yes or no) was used in the final analyses. To evaluate the potential impact of comorbidity, indicator variables for each type of prevalent condition were examined (i.e., MI, stroke, diabetes, hypertension, cancer, broken bones). Additional indicator variables were also included reflecting onset of any of these conditions during the 1988–1991 follow-up period.

Analyses

Data were analyzed using the Statistical Analysis System version 6.12 for Windows (SAS Institute, 1996) on personal computer. Univariate analyses were conducted first to examine basic statistical characteristics of all variables using PROC UNIVARIATE and PROC FREQ. Descriptive statistical analyses were conducted to estimate means and standard deviations (for continuous variables) and percentages (for dichotomous variables) for groups characterized by the presence of different chronic conditions. To test for relationships between baseline characteristics and changes in physical functioning, residualized change scores were examined—that is, change in functioning measured as the difference in functioning scores (1991 less 1988 baseline, adjusted for baseline physical functioning) (Menard, 1991). Multiple regression analyses with backward selection based on the full set of potential risk factors were conducted for each of the chronic condition groups (as well as the group without chronic conditions) to identify risk factors that made significant, independent contributions ($p \leq$ .05) to observed differences in patterns of change in physical functioning. Because analyses of change are subject to concern about the extent to which measured changes reflect real change or simply measurement error (e.g., regression to the mean or other unreliability effects), we also examined a series of logistic regression models where individuals in the bottom third (most negative) of all change scores were compared with everyone else. The criterion for defining "decline" was based on an adaptation of the Reliable Change Index developed by Hageman and Arrindell (1993, 1999). Using information on change scores and the reliability of those scores (calculated based on our test-retest reliability data for the physical functioning measure), a reliable change score is calculated, indicating whether an individual's change score can be reliably classified as *declined, improved,* or *no reliable evidence of change.* Logistic regression models were used to evaluate the extent to which the same factors seen in the linear regression models would be found to predict "decliners" versus others.

Examination of the potential impact of missing data yielded little evidence for such effects. At baseline, there was very little missing data (89% of cohort had complete data). Those excluded due to missing data on one or more variables had somewhat lower physical and cognitive functioning scores and were less likely to report any regular physical activity. There were no differences in exclusion rates based on the presence or absence of chronic conditions. For the longitudinal data, 81% of cohort had complete data. Those excluded due to missing data on 1991 physical functioning were more likely to be non-White and to have missing income information from baseline, and they also had poorer lung function at baseline. Mortality between 1988 and 1991 accounted for 22% of those with missing longitudinal outcome data.

Results

Table 5.1 presents descriptive information, showing the sociodemographic, health status, health behavior, social, and psychological char-

Table 5.1 Descriptive Baseline (1988) Data on Sociodemographic, Health Status, Behavioral, and Psychosocial Factors by Chronic Condition Groups

	No chronic conditions (N = 310)	History of hypertension (N = 563)	History of diabetes (N = 155)	History of cardiovascular (N = 154)	History of cancer (N = 213)	History of bone fracture (N = 291)
	M (SD)	M (SD)	M (SD)	M (SD)	M (SD)	M (SD)
Sociodemographic characteristics						
Age (70–79)	74.13 (2.68)	74.28 (2.74)	74.30 (2.70)	74.38 (2.84)	74.55 (2.74)	74.28 (2.68)
Gender (% male)	47.74	41.03	45.81	63.64*	43.19	32.75 **
Ethnicity (% black)	18.45	24.73*	20.13	12.34	9.43*	15.96
Annual household income (% ≥ 10,000/yr)	53.22	47.78	49.03	51.95	48.83	48.24
Education (% ≥ high school)	51.94	43.06**	38.06**	37.01 **	47.42	47.54
Health Status—1988						
Cognitive function (20–80)	53.19 (9.92)	52.41 (10.21)	51.29 (10.31)	52.00 (10.20)	54.78 (8.70)	53.09 (10.24)
Lung function (best peak flow; 30–710L/min)	388.17 (116.96)	376.93 (113.47)	401.10 (119.94)	401.58 (127.42)	383.81 (113.15)	355.70** (113.60)
Body mass index (14.5–43.9)	25.40 (4.04)	26.65 (4.40)*	27.22 (4.12)**	26.16 (3.77)*	26.07 (4.26)	25.57 (4.26)
Waist-hip ratio (0.55–1.19)	0.88 (0.09)	0.89 (0.08)	0.91 (0.07)**	0.91 (0.07)**	0.88 (0.08)	0.87 (0.08)
High DBP (%)	8.41	16.58**	7.14	7.95	11.79	13.12*
High SBP (%)	34.30	53.79**	48.05**	48.34**	33.65	38.30
Hx MI (%)	0	14.4***	13.0***	88.3***	13.6***	12.4***
Hx stroke (%)	0	2.8**	4.6***	19.0***	2.3**	3.4***
Hx HBP (%)	0	100.0***	60.6***	59.1***	47.9***	42.8***
Hx diabetes (%)	0	16.8***	100.0***	17.0***	10.3***	12.7***
Hx cancer (%)	0	18.2***	14.3***	20.9***	100.0***	20.6***
Hx fracture (%)	0	22.3***	24.0***	27.4***	28.2***	100.0***
Percentage of any medication use	55.2	68.6**	67.74**	64.3*	62.0	65.4*

Incident conditions—1988–1991						
MI (%)	1.9	2.5	4.5	0.60	2.3	1.4
Stroke (%)	1.6	3.4	5.8**	3.2	5.2*	3.4
HBP (%)	1.0	—	3.9*	1.3	1.9	1.4
Diabetes (%)	6.1	6.4	—	3.2	2.8	5.5
Cancer (%)	6.4	4.4	7.7	5.2	0**	5.8
Fracture (%)	4.2	2.7	0**	3.2	2.0	1.4*
Health behaviors						
Current smokers (%)	19.03	14.56	7.10**	10.39*	11.74*	16.20
Pack-years (0–78,093)	8941	7920	6458	12857	9569	8077
	(12,237)	(12,184)	(11,788)*	(16,039)*	(15,019)	(12,592)
Strenuous activity (kcal/wk) (0–160)	21.52	19.16	15.23	20.20	23.80	22.78
	(27.13)	(25.68)	(22.72)**	(29.72)	(27.59)	(26.10)
Moderate or strenuous activity (% any)	77.42	75.13	74.84	74.68	84.04	89.93
Ethyl alcohol (oz/month) (0–99.9)	4.31 (10.11)	3.13 (8.02)	2.27 (6.78)**	4.30 (9.15)	4.43 (8.94)	3.38 (8.76)
Social relationships						
Married (%)	50.65	45.81	59.09	52.29	45.07	34.86 **
Number of ties (0–30)	10.27 (5.00)	10.14 (5.39)	10.26 (5.22)	10.46 (5.41)	9.28 (4.87)*	9.90 (5.35)
Emotional support (0–3)	2.46 (0.55)	2.50 (0.51)	2.46 (0.50)	2.39 (0.54)	2.41 (0.58)	2.46 (0.57)
Instrumental support (0–3)	1.69 (0.77)	1.66 (0.72)	1.79 (0.74)**	1.70 (0.72)	1.48 (0.76)	1.60 (0.74)
Conflict or demands (0–3)	0.64 (0.60)	0.61 (0.55)	0.73 (0.58)	0.67 (0.60)	0.66 (0.57)	0.66 (0.60)
Psychological characteristics						
Self-efficacy beliefs						
Interpersonal efficacy (3–12)	9.53 (1.40)	9.17 (1.22)**	9.42 (1.28)	9.02 (1.32)**	9.23 (1.30)*	9.29 (1.36)*
Instrumental efficacy (7–16)	11.10 (1.29)	10.98 (1.16)	11.11 (1.15)	11.02 (1.16)	11.03 (1.25)	11.03 (1.23)
Total psychological symptomatology	63.46	65.94	64.93	67.23	67.31	66.46
(50–119)	(10.44)	(12.69)**	(11.32)**	(12.95)**	(12.96)**	(12.31)***

Note: Group comparisons reflect comparisons of each chronic condition group with those reporting no chronic conditions.
*p < 0.05, **p < 0.01, ***p < .001.

acteristics for each of the chronic condition groups as compared with those reporting no such conditions. As shown, those with prevalent chronic conditions differed from those reporting no chronic conditions with respect to sociodemographic, behavioral, and psychosocial characteristics. There were proportionately more men in the prevalent CVD group, while the fracture group had proportionately fewer men; the prevalent CVD group also had proportionally fewer subjects who completed high school, as do the HBP and diabetes groups. Those with a history of hypertension were significantly more likely to be African American while those with a history of cancer were significantly less likely to be African Americans.

Those with prevalent chronic conditions, particularly those with a history of high blood pressure, diabetes or prevalent CVD, also exhibited generally poorer health status and health behavior profiles than those with no reported conditions. Comorbidity patterns, however, were generally similar across the various disease groups, with hypertension being the most commonly reported other condition. Incidence of new conditions was generally low (6% or less).

In terms of health behaviors, those with CVD reported significantly greater pack-years of prior smoking, though they were less likely to be current smokers. By contrast, those with diabetes were less likely to be current smokers and reported significantly fewer pack-years of smoking; they also reported significantly less strenuous physical activity. Those with a history of cancer differed from those with no reported conditions only with respect to smoking status: They were less likely to be current smokers (though their reported pack-years of smoking tended to be higher, $p > .05$).

Differences across groups were also seen with regard to social and psychological characteristics. Those with no chronic conditions generally scored higher on psychological well-being (i.e., higher self-efficacy and lower psychological symptomatology). There were fewer differences, however, with respect to social network characteristics. Those with a history of cancer reported fewer social ties while those with a history of fracture were less likely to be married. There were no group differences with respect to reported levels of emotional support or levels of demands or conflicts and the only difference with respect to instrumental support was the higher reported levels of such support among diabetics.

With respect to our outcome of interest—physical functioning—those with no reported chronic conditions exhibited better physical functioning at baseline ($M = 2.85$, $SD = 0.45$) than those with a history of HBP, diabetes, CVD, or a history of fracture (see Table 5.2). Those reporting a history of diabetes and those with a history of fracture exhibited the poorest functioning ($M = 2.693$, $SD = 0.48$ and $M = 2.699$, $SD = 0.57$, respectively). With respect to patterns of change in physical functioning from 1988 to 1991, differences in mean change scores between groups with and without chronic conditions were generally not statistically significant, largely as a result of the considerable heterogeneity within groups in the patterns of change in functioning, a factor that is the focus of analyses reported below. The one exception was for diabetics: They exhibited the largest declines ($M = -0.121$, $SD = 0.55$) and these declines were significantly greater than those seen for the group with no conditions. Those with prevalent CVD exhibited the next largest declines ($M = -0.06$, $SD = 0.52$), followed by those with hypertension ($M = -0.047$, $SD = 0.52$), though these declines were not significantly different from that seen among those with no conditions.

Factors Affecting Longitudinal Patterns of Change

Stepwise, backward multiple regression analyses were conducted to identify factors associated with differences in patterns of change in physical functioning over a 2.5 year interval. For each of the disease groups (and those with no conditions), the full set of potential predictors were entered initially in each model; predictors with p $\leq$ 0.05 were retained in the final models (see Table 5.3). Among subjects with no prevalent conditions, those showing less decline were characterized by higher incomes, higher initial levels of cognitive functioning, absence of high systolic BP and better health habits as reflected by reports of engaging in some regular moderate and/or strenuous physical activity; these effects were independent of baseline physical functioning. Baseline physical functioning was also a predictor of decline: higher baseline functioning predicted greater decline by 1991.

Examination of the pattern of predictors for the five groups reporting prevalent chronic conditions at baseline revealed two notably consistent effects. One was the effect of initial levels of physical functioning, with higher initial physical functioning predicting greater decline at follow-up in all groups. The other consistent finding was the protective effect of regular physical activity for three of the five chronic condition groups. Among participants with prevalent CVD, those reporting greater amounts of regular strenuous activity show less decline

Table 5.2 Levels of Physical Functioning and Changes in Physical Functioning (1988 to 1991) by Chronic Condition Group

	Mean score of physical functioning (SD)					
	No chronic conditions (N = 254)	History of hypertension (N = 452)	History of diabetes (N = 125)	History of cardio-vascular disease (N = 119)	History of cancer (N = 172)	History of bone fracture (N = 230)
1988 performance	2.852 (0.45)	2.717 (0.53)***	2.693 (0.46)***	2.713 (0.57)*	2.805 (0.47)	2.699 (0.57)***
1991 performance	2.843 (0.57)	2.670 (0.63)***	2.572 (0.63)***	2.653 (0.71)**	2.850 (0.52)	2.686 (0.65)**
Change in performance (1991–1988 score)	−0.009 (0.48)	−0.047 (0.52)	−0.121 (0.55)*	−0.060 (0.52)	0.044 (0.48)	−0.013 (0.49)

*$p < 0.05$, **$p < .01$, ***$p < .001$ (when compared with those reporting no chronic conditions).

in functioning. Among those with HBP or a history of cancer, the dichotomous designation of *any* versus *no regular moderate or strenuous leisure activity* was associated with lower risks for decline.

The various prevalent condition groups show greater variation with respect to the sociodemographic, health status, social, and psychological factors that were related to change in physical functioning. Among those with hypertension, less decline was seen in younger individuals, those with better cognition and better lung function as well as lower BMI, and less reported conflict with others; use of medications was associated with better functioning. Not surprisingly, onset of conditions such as MI, stroke, or fracture was also associated with greater decline. Among diabetics, those showing less decline tended to be men and also reported use of medications. Diabetics with a history of fracture were more likely to decline. Like those with hypertension, diabetics reporting greater social conflict with others exhibited more decline over time. Among those with prevalent CVD, less decline was seen among those with better baseline lung function and those reporting greater emotional support from others. Incident fractures in this group were also marginally associated with greater declines (p = 0.06). Among those with a history of cancer, less decline was seen in those characterized by younger age, higher income, not smoking, and less alcohol consumption. Instrumental efficacy beliefs were also associated with less decline. Those reporting greater comorbidity (i.e., hypertension, diabetes, or fractures) were more likely to decline. Among those with a history of fracture, factors associated with less likelihood of decline in functioning included absence of high systolic BP or diabetes, and less psychological symptomatology at baseline.

Because analyses of change are subject to concern about the extent to which measured changes reflect real change or measurement error (e.g., regression to the mean or other unreliability effects), a series of logistic regression models were also examined. Individuals with change scores indicating "reliable decline" (i.e., those in approximately the bottom third of the change score distribution) were compared with everyone else to evaluate the extent to which the same factors seen in the earlier linear regression models would be found to predict "decliners." These analyses reveal a pattern of significant effects that largely parallels those from the linear regression models (data available on request from first author). For those reporting no chronic conditions, decliners are characterized by lower incomes and no regular physical activity. Among those with HBP, decliners were characterized by older age, worse lung function, and higher BMIs and also reported no reg-

Table 5.3 Multivariate Models Predicting Changes in Physical Performance from 1988 to 1991—Comparison of Sociodemographic, Health Status, Behavioral and Psychosocial Predictors Across the Chronic Condition Groups (Coefficients are reported only for factors with p-value < .10)[a]

	No chronic conditions (N = 227)	History of hypertension (N = 402)	History of diabetes (N = 116)	History of CVD (N = 107)	History of cancer (N = 155)	History of bone fracture (N = 212)
Sociodemographic characteristics	beta	beta	beta	beta	beta	beta
Age		−0.03**			−0.026*	
Gender (Male/Female)			0.19*			
Ethnicity (Af. Amer/White)						
Income						
(≥ $10K/yr vs < $10K/yr)	0.178**				0.229***	
Baseline health & functioning	beta	beta	beta	beta	beta	beta
Physical performance	−0.373***	−0.461**	−0.335**	−0.396**	−0.585***	−0.34***
Cognitive function	0.0075*	0.009***				
Lung fx (best peak flow)		0.001***		0.001**		
Body mass index		−0.019***				
High SBP (yes/no)						−0.20**
Hx. diabetes (yes/no)					−0.35***	
Hx fractures (yes/no)			−1.27**		−0.14*	−.24**
Medications (yes/no)		0.16**	0.27**			
Incident conditions (1988–1991)	beta	beta	beta	beta	beta	
MI (yes/no)		−0.39***				
Stroke (yes/no)		−0.33**				
Fracture (yes/no)		−0.28*				

Health behaviors					
Smoker (yes/no)					−0.23*
Strenuous activity (kcal/wk)	0.17*	0.13*		0.0034*	
Any moderate or strenuous Activity (yes/no)					0.35***
Alcohol (oz/month)					−0.001*
Social relationships					
Married (yes/no)					
Number of ties					
Emotional support				0.23**	
Instrumental support					
Conflict or demands		−0.095*	−0.152*		
Psychological characteristics					
Self-Efficacy Beliefs					
Interpersonal efficacy beliefs					
Instrumental efficacy beliefs					0.054*
Psychological symptomatology					−0.01**
Model R^2	0.16	0.24	0.22	0.19	0.42
F-test for overall model	6.97	11.43	6.22	4.89	9.52
p-value under F-test	0.0001	0.0001	0.0002	0.0005	0.0001

*.01 < p ≤ .05.
**.001 < p ≤ .01.
***p ≤ .001.

[a]Table presents results from the final step of a stepwise regression analysis for each of the groups indicated in the column headings. For each group, only factors that were significant at the .05 level or beyond were retained in the final model (shown by the presence of a coefficient listed under that column). If no coefficient is shown, that factor was not included in the final model for that group. Variables not listed in the table (i.e. education, waist-hip ratio, high DBP, Hx. hypertension, marital status, number of social ties, instrumental support and interpersonal efficacy beliefs) had no significant effect in any of the groups examined.

ular physical activity and more frequent social conflict; they are also more likely to have experienced an incident MI during follow-up. Within the group of diabetics, decliners were characterized by greater social conflict as well as the absence of medication use. For those with CVD, decliners are characterized by no reported regular physical activity and less frequent emotional support. Among those with a history of cancer, decliners are characterized by higher initial physical functioning and no reported regular physical activity. Among those with a history of fracture, decliners were characterized by higher systolic BP and more frequent social conflict with others.

Discussion

The analyses presented here examined the hypothesis that lifestyle behaviors and as sociodemographic and psychosocial factors influence patterns of change in physical functioning over time in groups of older adults with hypertension, diabetes, CVD, cancer, and/or fractures. Findings from these analyses suggest two significant points.

First, for those reporting no conditions and for three of the five "disease" groups, engaging in regular physical exercise was seen to exert a protective effect: Those who reported that they engaged in regular physical exercise were significantly less likely to experience declines over the 2.5–year follow-up. Only those with diabetes and fractures did not show this effect.

Second, social and psychological factors were unrelated to changes in functioning among those who report no chronic conditions at baseline. However, psychosocial factors did show significant, independent associations with change in functioning for individuals reporting the presence of HBP, diabetes, CVD, cancer, or fractures. For those with prevalent CVD, greater emotional support was a significant, independent predictor of less decline. Among those with HBP and diabetes, greater reported social conflict was associated with significantly greater risks for decline. Instrumental self-efficacy beliefs were protective against declines among those with a history of cancer, though this effect was seen only in the linear regression analyses (i.e., not in the logistic models that predict only more severe declines). For those with a history of fracture, lower levels of psychological symptomatology were associated with less risk of decline, though greater social conflict with others was associated with increased risks for decline.

We had not predicted these variations across disease groups with respect to the specific psychosocial factors that were found to be associated with patterns of change. Rather, our more general hypothesis had been that such psychosocial factors would influence patterns of change. Post hoc, it is possible to offer some suggestions as to the possible reasons for these observed variations. None of the psychosocial factors explained patterns of change in physical functioning among those with no chronic conditions at baseline. This is consistent with some earlier work from our group suggesting that such psychosocial factors may impact on change in functioning more strongly among more vulnerable groups (e.g., those with poorer health and lower socioeconomic status) Unger, McAvay, Bruce, Berkman, & Seeman, 1999). Thus, it may be that for individuals in relatively better health (i.e., those with no chronic conditions at baseline), psychosocial factors have less impact on changes in functioning. For this group, exercise was the only lifestyle factor seen to be a significant predictor of patterns of change in functioning.

That levels of emotional support were protective among those with prevalent CVD is also consistent with previous research indicating that such support is also protective against mortality among those with CVD (Berkman, Leo-Summers, & Horwitz, 1992; King, Reis, Porter, & Norsen, 1993; Krumholz et al., 1998). Possible explanations for these links between emotional support and mortality or functional decline include hypothesized buffering effects of such support to reduce the stress of dealing with a chronic condition (Lyons, Sullivan, & Ritvo, 1995). Support for this proposed pathway can be seen in recent evidence indicating that those reporting more emotional support exhibit lower levels of physiological arousal and that such lower arousal is linked to better outcomes, including lower mortality and better physical functioning (Seeman, Levy-Storms, Singer, & Ryff, in press; Seeman, Singer, Horwitz, McEwen, 1997).

The fact that social conflict was seen to be associated with declines in functioning among those with hypertension and diabetes could reflect the relatively greater demands on those individuals to manage the disease through lifestyle modifications (diet, exercise). If such modifications serve as a lightning rod for social conflict with other family members (e.g., family demands that the subject comply or criticism related to subject's need for special foods, etc.), then individuals with these conditions may be at greater risk for exposure to social conflict. Such conflict is seen to predict poorer functional outcomes and could reflect an association between conflict and poorer disease management or between conflict and greater general physiological arousal, which has been shown to predict poor functional outcomes (Seeman et al., 1997; Seeman et al., in press).

For those with cancer or fractures, more psychological characteristics were seen to predict patterns of change. One might speculate that in both cases, the relatively greater role of individual psychological characteristics (levels of instrumental efficacy for those with cancer and levels of psychological symptomatology for those with fractures) may reflect a greater tendency for these two types of conditions to have more direct impacts on functioning as a result of surgery or chemotherapy. In these cases, the individual's psychological outlook may impact significantly on the degree to which they work to recover or maintain higher levels of functioning. Given the post hoc nature of the explanations offered for the observed pattern of psychosocial influences within the different disease groups, further research is obviously needed to evaluate their validity.

In considering these results, it is important to acknowledge some potential limitations of the data. Foremost is the question of the generalizeability of the findings presented here. As indicated at the outset, the MacArthur cohort was selected in 1988 (baseline) to represent the top third of those aged 70 to 79 with respect to physical and cognitive functioning. Thus, our results may not generalize to the broader population of older adults. This is a question that will need to be addressed by further research. A related issue concerns the fact that the MacArthur study database contains information only on the presence of chronic conditions; there is no information on the diagnosed severity of these conditions. Thus, it was not possible to examine of whether factors found to predict differences in functioning within groups were equally influential for those with more severe versus milder levels of disease. Strengths of the reported analyses, however, include the fact that the MacArthur cohort reflects considerable diversity with respect to gender, ethnicity, and socioeconomic status, and the rich array of potential health status, health behavior, and social and psychological factors that were assessed and available for consideration as potential predictors of functioning.

The findings reported here highlight the fact that levels of functioning among older adults with chronic conditions are not solely determined by health status. This is noteworthy because despite considerable and important research and clinical efforts to reduce risks for various chronic conditions, older age continues to be associated with increasing risks for most chronic conditions. Our findings also highlight the fact that levels of physical functioning in older adults who experience such chronic conditions are not immutably tied to these health conditions. Rather, levels of functioning and, importantly, patterns of change in functioning over time, were found to be influenced by potentially modifiable factors—physical exercise, social support, self-efficacy beliefs, and psychological symptomatology—independent of the presence of chronic conditions or other aspects of health status and of differences in sociodemographic characteristics. These findings suggest the potential utility, even among those with existing chronic conditions, of efforts to encourage regular physical activity in older adults as a means of promoting optimal levels of physical functioning. The data on the impact of social support and psychological profiles on patterns of change in functioning also suggest the potential utility of interventions in at risk older adults with chronic conditions (i.e., those reporting low levels of social support, a low sense of self-efficacy, and high levels of psychological symptomatology).

Though older adults are certainly likely to continue to experience greater risks for various chronic conditions, the findings reported here suggest that the functional consequences of such conditions can be significantly and positively influenced by various lifestyle factors—factors that are themselves potential targets for interventions to promote more optimal levels of functioning. Such evidence will hopefully serve to dispel perceptions of chronic conditions as harbingers of inevitable decline. Rather, evidence that lifestyle and psychosocial factors impact on functional status can hopefully serve to encourage the view that there are steps that can be taken to protect against functional declines, even in the face of chronic conditions.

Acknowledgments

Work on this chapter was supported by a grant from the AARP Andrus Foundation, by grants from the NIA (AG-17056, AG-17265), and by the MacArthur Research Network on Successful Aging and the MacArthur Research Network on SES and Health through grants from the John D. and Catherine T. MacArthur Foundation.

Chapter 6

Health Expectancy, Risk Factors, and Physical Functioning

Janice Penrod and Peter Martin

Typically the notion of successful aging in older adulthood conjures up images of individuals or groups of older adults who manage to avoid risk factors, function at an optimal physical level, and live long, healthy lives. Yet the impact of aging and adaptation involves more than risk factors and health, as becomes apparent when reading the previous chapters by Crimmins, Kim, and Hagedorn, and Seeman and Chen. Their two studies yield important insights that contribute to a fuller appreciation of the phenomenon of successful aging in the face of chronic conditions. In this chapter, we first address how these studies advance our understanding of successful aging and adaptation, followed by a discussion of conceptual issues that help to refine the potential for meaningful contribution to this growing body of knowledge. We begin with a discussion of the contribution made by Crimmins et al.

Crimmins and her colleagues aptly introduce the shifting markers of successful aging from a demographic perspective. As life expectancy increased dramatically during the twentieth century, mortality became a key marker of successful aging. Simply put, those who aged successfully lived; those who did not died. Although useful for defining population characteristics, this crude measure of successful aging revealed little about the characteristics of survivors. Such a perspective provided an understanding of demographic trends in mortality and life expectancy, yet it provided little insight into the quality of extended life.

An important question of any life expectancy measure concerns the level of analysis. We are reminded that life expectancy measures typically call for population-based definitions about what is successful and what is not. The term *life expectancy* itself is based on population projections, not on individual assessments. If the cohort born in 1994 had an average life expectancy of 75.7 years, then we learn something about the cohort just born, but we learn little about the chances that a particular baby born in 1994 will live to the year 2070.

Quality of Life and Successful Aging

The same issue is relevant for health expectancy measures. It is the health of a population that is typically discussed, not the health of individuals. Because of large-population estimates, it is difficult to imagine meaningful measures concerning the quality of life. An interest in *quality* of life emerged as a powerful partner to length of life as indicators of successful aging. This shift in perspective was a critical turn toward a better understanding of successful aging, especially as issues of increasing the length of *healthy* life were integrated into the U.S. national health goals. Knowing that most people live with multiple chronic conditions in later life, quantity of life (reflected in life expectancy rates) was ineffective for evaluating the quality of life experienced through this extended life span. Therefore, the notion of health expectancy (or years spent without significant disability or poor health) was developed to address this issue.

The definition of health expectancy employed in this and in other studies poses potential limitations on the utility of the work. For example, is health best captured by absence of morbidity (not a common state for most older adults), functional losses (despite available support systems), or states of disability (with limiting definitional issues)? While the operational definition of quality of life (i.e., health) assumed in many demographic studies is often limited by the availability of population-based data, the conceptual stance assumed by researchers reveals important perspectives that demand the reader's close attention.

Crimmins and colleagues (see chapter 4) assume the perspective that health is reflected in the number of years lived without severe, long-term disability or without disease. Disability is further defined as an inability "to perform personal care [i.e., activities of daily living] . . . and tasks necessary for independent living [i.e., instrumental activities of daily living]." Life without disease is operationally defined as the absence of the nine highly prevalent chronic conditions of older adulthood. An overall assessment of personal health is used further to provide a more comprehensive evaluation of the older adult's state of health. Given available population-based data, this perspective captures the phenomenon of health and aging not only through the presence of conditions but also through the impact of those conditions on everyday life. However, this perspective remains limited by an emphasis on physical wellness rather than on more holistic measures of the subjective quality of life.

It is interesting to note that "health expectancy" was not the first term used to describe a high quality of life.[1] First, the term *disability-free life expectancy* was used to focus on the absence of disabilities. A life with some disability, however, does not necessarily imply a life without quality. Consider a person whose mobility is restricted but who enjoys family life, volunteers for a phone bank, and manages most activities of their daily living. This person would not necessarily have a poor life quality. Perhaps because of this discrepancy, the term *active life expectancy* came into usage. Rather than focusing on disabilities, it seemed important to assess whether individuals could remain active and stay autonomous by effectively managing their activities of daily living.

The problem with this terminology turned out to be that "activity" might be defined in very different ways. In population studies assessing life expectancies, it typically refers to activities of daily living (i.e., the extent to which one can manage one's daily life). In studies of successful aging, however, it typically relates to a larger, less well-defined construct: an actively engaged person (see Kahn, chapter 3). Although Crimmins et al. use the term *health expectancy,* their assessment includes all three aspects mentioned above: (a) activity, defined as activity of daily living (i.e., the ability to perform personal care or routine needs); (b) disability, defined as the inability to perform ADL tasks; (c) health, defined as self-assessments of health (i.e., *good* or *better*) and by specific diseases, such as heart disease and arthritis. These alternative definitions turn out to be of paramount importance. Using the first criterion—activity of daily living—one can expect to

---

[1]Eileen Crimmins pointed out that there has been a long-standing debate about appropriate terminology. The term *disability-free life expectancy* seemed more limiting. The term *health expectancy* (or *health-adjusted life expectancy* as proposed by WHO) is a more generic term.

live 74.3 out of 75.7 years without impairment (considering the ability to perform personal care tasks). Using the second criterion— disability, one would expect only 62.1 years without disability. With regard to health, 66 years are expected to be in good or better subjective health. Finally, health expectancy is low when arthritis is the major criterion (i.e., 63.5 years) or high if diabetes is of concern (i.e., 72.5 years). Taken together, these results suggest that careful attention needs to be paid to the specific definition of health expectancy. Results support both the hypothesis of morbidity compression and the hypothesis of greater burden and disability (Fries & Crapo, 1981; Guralnik & Schneider, 1987; also see Seeman et al., chapter 5). The message to policy makers is two-sided: quality of life is high, except for the last year of life, if personal care is the criterion; or the message might be that older adults suffer from a long period of chronic diseases, on average 13.6 years, if any disability (most often arthritis) is considered as the main criterion for quality of life.

Measuring Health Expectancy Across Populations

Definitions of health expectancy also call for the assessment of measurement equivalence across subgroups of the population and over time (Schaie & Hofer, 2001). For example, would a measure of health expectancy for women be different than a health expectancy measure for men? Gender differences obtained in health research are often compelling, but are the differences really mean differences, or do men and women merely have differential views of health? The same could be said for ethnicity, social status, or other population categories. Furthermore, measurement equivalence over time is important to consider. Does the concept of health change over individual and historical time? What we consider to be a healthy lifestyle in midlife is not necessarily a healthy lifestyle in very old age (Forette, 1999). In order to track health expectancy changes over time, it is important to come to a unified standard of what health expectancy is and how to measure it consistently across populations and time. Such a standard would also help with health expectancy comparisons across nations and cultures. It is therefore important to develop a robust international measure of health expectancy.

Another caveat to this theoretical interpretation of available data is that the data available through the National Health Interview Surveys (NHIS) rely on *reported* prevalence and functional capability, a report that, in fact, may be offered by proxy respondents (Schoeni, Freedman, &Wallace, 2001). This method of reporting calls into question the validity or truth-value of the proxy's perceptions of the older adult's need for the help of other persons to complete ADLs and IADLs versus the perception of the older adult, or even versus observed ratings of the same.

A further limitation of the NHIS data set is the exclusion of institutionalized and military populations. Institutional populations typically are thought to refer to those in nursing homes; however, the definitional boundaries of institutionalization employed by this national survey calls into question those residing in assisted living facilities as well (Schoeni et al., 2001). The U.S. Bureau of the Census (1997) defines institutions by using characteristics of group quarters and restricted ability of movement in and out of the facility. The exclusion of the nursing home population, although large in number and high in incidence of disease and disability, actually has little impact on overall trends because it only represents about 5% of the population over age 65. However, the possible exclusion of assisted living facilities poses a more interesting dilemma, in that approximately 1 million older adults with varying health conditions and degrees of disablement reside in these facilities (see Rakowski, Clark, Miller, & Berg, chapter 2).

The trends projected by Crimmins, Kim, and Hagedorn (chapter 4) reveal important insights about the length of healthy and unhealthy life according to the indicators discussed above. These findings challenge the notion that old age is fraught with disability. For example, at age 65, of the 17.4 years of life expectancy, 10.5 years are estimated to be lived "disability free." Of the disabled years, most will be spent requiring assistance with IADL tasks, not the more severe disability posed by ADL restrictions. Gender differences reveal that the life expectancy of men at age 65 is different than that of women. Though men are projected to live fewer years in total, they experience an earlier onset of need for assistance with a markedly shorter duration. Similarly, race differences highlight disparities in both the quality and length of years in later life.

Estimates of health expectancy, of course, are based on means, rather than on the distribution around the mean. Although mean values provide us with a good intuitive sense of expected life-span health, it would be important to know what proportion of the population falls into a narrow band around the mean, and what proportion of the population could be found with a lower health expectancy or higher life expectancy.

Regarding living with disability, Crimmins and her colleagues note that the subjective state of health assessment reveals that the onset of disability does not correspond to health ratings of *less than good*. This finding reinforces the notion that loss of IADL or even ADL capability does not directly impact older adults' personal assessment of health status. The basis of this notion remains questionable. Do these adults expect such limitations as a function of aging? Is there a lag in changing one's consciousness to face such changes? Or are support systems more responsive to early needs but somehow change over time, decreasing in their effectiveness for supporting the older adult?

The significance of the work by Crimmins et al. is that it begins to clarify not only quantity of life, but also the quality of those extended years. Though this work does not address the nuances of the individual's trajectory of disability, it is an important contribution. The focus on chronic conditions captures the nature of health in the later years of life, yet questions about the interaction of chronicity with acute episodes remain unanswered. Projections of years of life lived in states of disability versus healthy years are enlightening on a large scale, but do not tell us how those years occur. Kahn asserts that physical capabilities change over time, creating short-term periods of disablement. Although disability need not be a permanent state in the individual's life trajectory, the effects of short-term events on population-based demographics remain unclear. Can we expect the years of disability to be compressed at the end of life, or are there more sporadic periods of gains and declines (perhaps in relation to acute episodes superimposed on preexisting chronicity)? Finally, how does the adequacy of support systems affect a more qualitative perspective of quality of life for those who require assistance?

Changing Our Thinking About Aging

Health policy and large-scale program planning rely on an understanding of critical demographic issues as a basis for decision-making. This work signifies an important shift toward attending not only to the years of life achieved by survivors (life expectancy), but also to the health status enjoyed across those years (health expectancy). It marks an important conceptual turn in how we think about aging in the aggregate sense. Continued exploration of issues surrounding quantity and quality of extended years in population aging is crucial to refining the potential contribution of this understanding.

The implications of differential health expectancy for health policies are profound. Does the differential assessment of population subgroups mean that health policies should target disadvantaged groups? Should women receive differential health benefits than men? Should disadvantaged groups based on ethnicity and social class obtain differential health benefits to increase their health expectancy? What is the role of education in predicting a long and healthy life? Perhaps early education plays an important role in establishing healthy lifestyle patterns. But what are the chances that health interventions in midlife or later life would impact health expectancy?[2] The timing of "third" variables, such as education, income, or other resources is therefore important to consider. Are people who have disadvantages in early childhood disadvantaged for the rest of their lives? Can education, income, and other resources be compensated for at a later time? It seems that much work needs to be done to move toward differential health expectancy and differential timing so that policy decisions can be made. One way to learn more about differential predictors is to assess risk and protective factors for optimal functioning, a topic that was the focus of the study by Seeman and Chen, presented in chapter 5, which we now consider.

Seeman and Chen's Study on Physical Decline

Seeman and Chen focus on a more limited sample (the MacArthur studies) to derive an analysis of the impact of selected factors on declines in physical functioning over a 2.5–year time span. Although Crimmins et al. conceptualized the presence of chronic conditions as a precursor to states of disability, Seeman and Chen questioned this assumption as they evaluated whether or not the presence of multiple conditions was associated with decline in functioning, given the influence of within-group variation in relation to key lifestyle and psycho-

---

[2]Robert Kahn elaborated on the "power of education." He suggested that future work may consider two separate paths: The first obvious one suggests that education improves health behavior because people who become sophisticated early in life live their whole lives by making health-promotive behavioral choices. The second path, not in conflict with the first one, suggests that education may merely be a surrogate for socioeconomic status. More highly educated people live in different neighborhoods, are exposed to different environmental hazards, and make different choices than less educated people. It would therefore be useful to find out to what extent education effects persist, even if we can introduce controls for income, or whether most of the effect operates through income.

social characteristics. Their research focus required a different data set for the analysis, one that provided measures of an extended panel of variables over time. The clear strength of Seeman and Chen's study is that it takes into account changes in physical functioning rather than merely one-time assessments.

Seeman and Chen used data from the MacArthur Studies of Successful Aging for their investigation. The sample size and variety of available measures makes this sample especially appropriate for the inquiry. The data set allows longitudinal analysis of individuals rather than group trending and controls for measurement error versus real change.

The MacArthur Studies of Successful Aging provided necessary data, but it is limited to relatively high-functioning older adults, aged 70 to 79. The data set includes a wide range in other variables, for example, socioeconomic status. The conditions selected for study included hypertension, diabetes, cardiovascular disease, cancer, and broken bones. Though the population prevalence rates support the inclusion of these conditions, it is important to note that selection was driven by prevalence rates reported in the data set; that is, there were large enough numbers to enable analysis. It would be important to examine these results in light of other types of chronic conditions, for example, arthritis or osteoporosis without fracture.

Although many of the older adults experienced comorbidity (i.e., more than one chronic condition), subjects were classified into multiple disease groups for reported conditions. Analyses focused on all subjects reporting each condition. One caveat of the Seeman and Chen study is that limited sample size precluded an analysis of the effects of comorbidity. For example, hypertension was the most commonly reported comorbid condition yet, those with hypertension demonstrated an association between social conflict and significantly greater risks for decline. The potential confounding effect of living with multiple conditions is not accounted for in this association. Since comorbidity is a common phenomenon among older adults (for example, see Poon et al., chapter 7), the effects of co-occurring conditions warrant further consideration in subsequent studies. Though these authors do report that those experiencing greater comorbidity were more likely to decline, the complexities of comorbidity remain fruitful ground for research designed to deepen our understanding of the health status of older adults.

The study reported by Seeman and Chen methodically addressed multiple variables using a comprehensive battery of measures. The focus of examining change over time on the level of the individual is a significant strength of the study, for it provides insights regarding intra-individual changes rather than group means. Such insights are especially valuable given the researchers' sensitive approach to standard variables, for example, examining negative consequences of conflictive social support and including both work and leisure activities in their assessment of physical functioning. Their study provides plausible post hoc analyses and interpretation that reliably reflect real change rather than potential effects of measurement error.

The results of the Seeman et al. study also make theoretical and conceptual contributions. The finding that higher incomes and higher levels of cognitive functioning predict lower decline suggests that psychosocial resources play a prominent role in the maintenance of good health. Other studies have proposed that individual and socio-economic resources are salient predictors of, and mediators between, lifelong stress and physical health (Martin, in press). It would be desirable to develop and test more elaborate resource models that would predict differing levels of health, or more generally successful aging. Such models appear to be more common for health habits, another important set of predictors in the Seeman et al. study. Health belief models have commonly been used to test the effect of healthy life styles on physical outcomes (Leventhal, Rabin, Leventhal, & Burns, 2001; Rosenstock, Strecher, & Becker, 1988). In particular, the effect of exercise appears to gain status as an important protective function (Blair et al., 1995; Hakim et al., 1998).

Perhaps most important, Seeman and Chen aptly argue that health status is not "immutably tied" to the presence of certain health conditions. Rather, "the findings here suggest that the functional consequences of such conditions can be significantly and positively influenced by various lifestyle factors." The identification of modifiable risk factors that may enable interventions to change the course of health in aging is a significant contribution to this literature.

What These Studies Tell Us

What do these studies tells us about successful aging? It is important to recognize that demographic studies of late life necessarily capture the experiences of *survivors*. Those who did not age "successfully" died before they reached an age of interest for late-life demographic trends. This is not a new notion; it is simply a function of population-based studies of late life. However, a closer examination of the assumptions of what comprises successful aging does reveal interesting insights.

First, consider Rowe and Kahn's three criteria for successful aging: avoid disease and disability, maintain physical and mental function, and be actively engaged in life. Though the assessment of engagement in life cannot be derived from the operational definitions used by Crimmins et al., their focus on disease as disability as reflected in basic and higher order functional demands rings true to the conceptual frame proposed by Rowe and Kahn (1997). One may even assert that the subjective assessment of personal health may reflect active engagement with life (at least to a degree deemed acceptable to the older adult respondent).

The MacArthur Studies of Successful Aging, as discussed by Seeman and Chen, defines "success" (in aging) as no ADL deficit and not more than one mobility or physical performance deficit. These criteria actually may be less stringent than the criteria on which the NHIS data set is based (a "need for help" with ADL and IADL activities). Yet other important criteria, such as avoidance of disease and disability, require further investigation.

Schmidt's definition of successful aging, as cited by Strawbridge and Wallhagen (see chapter 1) allows for minimal disruption of usual function, even though signs and symptoms of chronic illness may be present. Despite the fact that this perspective is quite applicable to common health states of older adults, consider the difference in the conceptual frame of successful aging posed by this view versus that of Crimmins and colleagues. Strawbridge and Wallhagen (chapter 1) interpret Schmidt as allowing for "a little difficulty," while the Crimmins' study is based on a criterion of "needing help with" activities. Are these measures of successful (or healthy) aging based on conceptually congruent criteria, or could the "little difficulties" with which many older adults coexist prompt a positive response to a question based on a "need for help"? Once again, the conceptual clarity of successful aging becomes an issue. Perhaps, the perspective of Seeman and Chen's investigation of real change over time, without focusing specifically on the number or presence of conditions or on the need for assistance, provides the most cogent perspective of successful aging on the level of the individual.

Rakowski et al. (see chapter 2) propose that other dimensions of "successful aging" be addressed by its conceptualization. They assert that parameters of successful aging must accommodate those who live with multiple illnesses *and* those who have functional impairments, and that definitions of successful aging should not create a dichotomous categorization of others as unsuccessful at aging. Linguistics aside, Crimmins handled the NHIS data set to disentangle the presence of selected illnesses from the limitations that were used as defining characteristics of disability. Seeman and Chen challenge the assumption that the presence of conditions is indicative of inevitable decline. Conceptually, such distinctions reveal movement toward a more holistic conceptualization of what successful aging may mean.

But this congruence is lost when Baltes and Baltes' conceptualization of successful aging as "selective optimization with compensation" (Baltes & Baltes, 1990a) is applied. We suspect that older adults surveyed through the NHIS were healthy in some selected health domains, but we do not know how they optimized their health or whether they managed to compensate for any disability. We do not know the degree or effectiveness of support systems when the question stem prompts a response regarding "a need for help" versus compensation capability. Further, optimization cannot be captured in years lived with disease or years lived with disability. Seeman and Chen's comprehensive examination of lifestyle factors and individual change over time begins to reveal some elements of optimization, for example, physical activity patterns.

If optimization is related to context, as asserted by Rakowski et al., successful aging equals managing or balancing the demands of life with the capabilities of the individual, supported by whatever resources or assets are available to older adults. The Crimmins study measures demands posed by chronic illness and disability (as reflected in functional limitations) but fails to capture the more dynamic state of supported capability. Seeman and Chen address a range of variables that reflect resources and capability indirectly. Our work (Penrod et al., chapter 9) takes us one step closer to understanding this dynamic state of supported capability as the older adults revealed how the demands of comorbidity and related disablement were managed to maximize capability in everyday life.

Thus, the concept of successful aging remains rather nebulous. Each disciplinary perspective included in this text reveals something about the nature of this state of being, but we have yet to define accurately this high-order concept. Multiple perspectives of this complex reality appear to offer the most promise for understanding. Subjective reports of older adults and their significant others provide insights but often prematurely narrow the inquiry and, in turn, narrow the utility of the theoretical insights. Objective measures of capability within a range of demands yields yet another perspective of the realities of successful aging. But when these observations are subsequently interpreted through disciplinary lenses that define "normal" versus "successful" aging, the findings are again limited in their utility for enhancing a conceptual understanding of the phenomenon of interest.

Though some argue for a triangulation of findings related to successful aging, embracing multiple perspectives simply may be more feasible and more realistic, given the state of this science. Triangulation, as in surveying, relies on one's ability to focus on one point from at least two perspectives to assess convergence (and, therefore, increase the truth value of findings). When it comes to successful aging, it appears that the degree of incongruence in current conceptualizations may prohibit agreement on which point we should triangulate. The challenge to merge the life experience of successful aging, or perhaps aging *well*, with the scientific construct representing this complex phenomenon has certainly not been resolved. At best, we have begun to reveal the multiple realities surrounding this multifaceted concept.

Chapter 7

Coping with Comorbidity

Leonard W. Poon, Lynn Basford, Clare Dowzer, and Andrew Booth

I t is not uncommon for adults 65 and older to have three, four, five, or more coexisting health problems (Brody & Kleban, 1983; Guralnik, 1996). These problems, individually or in combination, can consume tremendous amounts of financial, physical, and psychological resources. In extreme cases, these problems are so overwhelming that a person does not have resources left to deal with anything else in his or her life. For most older people, these multiple health conditions are annoyances, and for many pose a serious threat to their continued function and independence. Satisfactory coping strategies for dealing with these problems would therefore greatly enhance the quality of their life.

A letter to the late newspaper columnist Ann Landers illustrates the impact of a chronic health condition on the well-being of one woman:

> Dear Ann Landers:
> I am a 45–year-old woman who has arthritis. Please print this list of "Do's and Don'ts" for dealing with a person who has this disease. Most folks don't have a clue. You would not believe the ignorance I have encountered.
> *Don't* assume because I look well that I feel well. Looks can be very deceiving. Many days I look great, but I feel terrible.
> *Don't* tell me you know how I feel. No one knows how anyone feels. Two people with the same disease may feel totally different. We all have varying thresholds of pain, and pain cannot be measured.

Don't tell me about your great-aunt Gertrude and her arthritis and how well she managed in spite of it. I am not Aunt Gertrude, and I am doing my best.

Don't tell me, "it could be worse." Yes, it could be, but I don't need to be reminded.

Don't decide what I am capable of doing. Arthritis doesn't affect the brain. Allow me to decide what activities I can participate in. There may be times I might make the wrong decision, and if I do, I'll know soon enough.

Don't be upset that you cannot ease my pain. It won't do any good for both of us to be miserable.

Don't ask me how I feel unless you really want to know. You may hear a lot more than you are prepared to listen to.

Don't assume because I did a certain activity yesterday that I can do it today. Arthritis is ever-changing.

Don't tell me about the latest fad "cure." I want to be cured more than anything, and if there is a legitimate cure out there, my doctor will let me know.

Do learn everything you can about the disease. The more you know, the better equipped you will be to know what to expect.

Do realize I am angry and frustrated with the disease, not with you.

Do let me know you are available to help me when I ask. I'll be grateful.

Do offer me lots of hugs and encouragement.

Do understand why I cancel plans at the last minute. I never know from one day to the next how I feel. Arthritis is like that.

Do continue to invite me to all the activities. Just because I am not able to bike ride along with the gang does not mean I can't meet you for the picnic at the end of the trail. Please let me decide.

Joy in Texas

"Joy in Texas," at age 45, is by no means an older adult by gerontology's definition. As revealed by this letter, however, arthritis can impact an individual physically, emotionally, and more importantly, by compromising her self-esteem and self-worth. Her situation raises many unanswered questions. What would be the impact if she had other health conditions (for example, a stroke) that could also influence her cognitively? Would this further impair or compound her ability to cope? What would be the impact if she were 65 or 70 instead of 45 years old? What would be the impact if she had other physical disabilities? How would the severity of each chronic disease influence her coping? And how would age, number and types of comorbidity, and severity of individual diseases increase the challenges of her coping?

Although there has been extensive study on health coping by older adults (e.g., Aldwin, Sutton, Chiara, & Spiro, 1996; Lehr & Kruse, 1992; McCrae, 1999; Moos & Mertens, 1999; Pearlman & Uhlmann, 1988), there is limited literature on how older adults cope with *multiple* health conditions. Therefore, the goals of our project on coping with multiple health conditions were twofold. During phase 1, we conducted an extensive literature search on coping with comorbidity and best practices of coping strategies for older adults. The purpose of phase 2 was to validate these strategies, using focus group methodologies. This chapter summarizes the findings of our literature search on coping with comorbidity in older adults, including the lessons we learned. Chapter 8 by Basford, Poon, Dowzer, and Booth focuses on the literature on older adults coping with 12 specific diseases. In chapter 9, Penrod, Gueldner, and Poon describe and discuss our findings from focus groups conducted with older adults in assisted living settings, who shared with us their health problems and coping strategies.

Literature Search Methodology

Data were collected for phase 1 of this study, using the worldwide research and clinical literature search methods and networks for best clinical practices developed by the International Cochran Collaboration (National Health Services Centre for Reviews and Dissemination [NHSCRD] 1996). The search was conducted under the auspices of the School of Health and Related Research and the School of Nursing at the University of Sheffield, United Kingdom. Details of this search can be found in a report by Dowzer, Basford, Booth, and Poon (1999). Twelve health conditions were selected for the literature search, based on mortality, morbidity, and patterns of disabilities among older adults. These conditions are as follows: cardiovascular disease, stroke and hypertension, respiratory diseases, diabetes, arthritis; colon, breast, lung, and prostate cancer; osteoporosis and fractures, and visual and hearing impairments. Two major research questions were posed for the literature search.

1. How do these conditions independently and in combination impact the physical, cognitive, and affective well-being of older individuals?
2. Which strategies have been shown in the research and clinical literature to be effective in coping with the conditions?

Twelve databases were searched, netting 7,139 studies; of these, 483 data-based papers were selected and reviewed. The following is a summary of our understanding of the literature, outlined in this chapter in five sections: (a) We begin with basic definitions of comorbidity and attempt to identify the complexities in defining and understanding it, as well as potential confounds and barriers that have impeded clear understanding of coping with comorbidity; (b) we then consider the impact of comorbidity on the quality of life of older adults and examine the dynamic nature of coping and comorbidity from individual, social-contextual, and disease-oriented perspectives; (c) we then provide an extensive summary of the effectiveness of cognitive, affective, physical, and combined strategies of coping in specific situations, based on published studies; (d) we present a review of coping strategies used in specific diseases, and (e) we summarize the fruits of our literature search on how older adults cope with comorbidity.

Definitions of Comorbidity and Barriers to Understanding Coping

In the case of "Joy in Texas," the literature tells us that in addition to her physically disabling arthritis, she may also experience bouts of depression. Further, she was told by her doctor that she has high blood pressure. The coexistence of three types of disease conditions is generally defined as *comorbidity*. However, two issues relating to the definition of comorbidity are not well articulated in the literature. First, do coexisting health conditions need to be similar in origin or etiology in order to be termed comorbidity; and second, should comorbidity be defined by the sum of the clinical manifestations or by the functions limited by the diseases? Such variations in the definition of comorbidity have contributed to differences in methods of measurement that continue to present a barrier to understanding the experience of coping with comorbidity.

Feinstein (1970) defined comorbidity as an associated illness arising from other diseases. He later referred to comorbidity as "any distinct additional clinical entity that has existed or that may occur during the clinical course of a patient who has the index disease under study" (Feinstein, 1970, p. 456). This definition is restrictive, in that it could exclude health conditions that have been misidentified, or those that may have been present in a prediagnosed state. In contrast, Guralnik (1996) employed the notion of aggregate score in the summation of conditions; that is, there may be a ceiling effect in the use of indices whereby the addition of other symptoms may be negligible once a certain aggregate score has been reached. Others have used a broader definition of comorbidity to include any disease, condition, malfunction, injury symptom, or syndrome that might attract medical attention (Kraemer, 1995). Thus, much of the discussion of comorbidity in the literature is how to define its scope. At present, however, it is fair to state that the coexistence of any two or more health conditions would be defined as comorbidity.

Variations in definition and focus have also led to differences in the measurement of the impact of comorbidity on outcomes (e.g., Charlson, Pompei, Ales, & MacKenzie, 1987; Greenfield, Apolone, McNeil, & Cleary, 1993; Linn, Linn, & Gurel, 1968). But the criticism of Rothenberg et al., (1997) was that many of the original methods of measuring comorbidity were developed by using of data from medical records. Variations in the reliability and validity of these instruments could be due to omission of relevant diagnoses, inappropriate inclusion of non-relevant information, and inappropriate weighting of conditions. The severity of a specific illness is recognized as important in the weighting of coexisting conditions to define comorbidity. Nonetheless, there are presently no satisfactory methods that take into account the relative impact of coexisting conditions and their severity (Guralnik, 1996; Charlson et al., 1987).

Two practical matters are noted in the assessment of comorbidity in everyday life. First, medical specialists tend to treat coexisting health conditions that are within their specialty and either ignore or leave the other conditions for others to treat (Van den Akker, Buntinx, & Knottnerus, 1996). This inconsistency in attention leads to differences in the quality of care of patients with similar comorbidity. Second, the patient's perception of the impact of coexisting conditions may be an important factor in how they deal with these conditions in everyday life.

This conceptual discussion relates to our question of whether co-morbidity should be defined by the collective clinical manifestations, or by the real or perceived functional impact of these conditions by the individual, or by both. We believe that an understanding of the perceived everyday impact of illness is important in the study of coping and the effectiveness of coping. Take for example the coexisting conditions of arthritis, depression, and hypertension being experienced by "Joy in Texas." Her nagging complaints dwelled on her arthritis because it has affected her functionally. Depression, on the other hand, would affectively impact her ability to cope with the arthritis. Both of these conditions have functional significance. The impact of hypertension on everyday function would be slight unless the severity is high. Joy would perceive a hierarchical ranking of impact from these three conditions and might cope accordingly, while a general practitioner might very likely treat these conditions equally. Coping strategies employed by Joy on these three coexisting conditions could very well be different from the treatment regimens recommended by her doctor.

Comorbidity Quality of Life of Older Adults

The co-occurrence of chronic conditions is more common among the older population (DeMaria & Cohen, 1987; Verbrugge, Lepkowski, & Imanaka, 1989). Also, Guralnik et al. (1993) reported an increase in the reporting of two or more chronic health conditions, from 50% among women 60 years or older to 70% among women 80 and older. In a Dutch general practice population, Van den Akker, Buntinx, Metsemakers, Roos, and Knottnerus (1998) reported a prevalence of multimorbidity of about 10% in those 19 years of age or younger, and up to 78% among those 80 years of age and older.

An increasing number of chronic conditions is associated with increasing frailty. With aging, there is an increasing loss of muscle mass and strength, decreased postural control, deconditioning, and altered immune responsiveness. Organs become less efficient and energy levels decline. The accumulation of chronic conditions magnifies their impact on physical, functional, and mental health (Angel & Angel, 1995). Severe and prolonged chronic health conditions often result in pain and suffering, disability, increasing difficulty with activities of daily living and the instrumental activities of daily living, and loss of independence (Fried & Guralnik, 1997). These continuing losses may severely compromise an individual's quality of life. Hence, successful coping with comorbidity is paramount to the quality of life of older adults.

Knottnerus et al. (1992) coined the phrase "social prevalence," meaning that more people are involved with the disease than just the patients themselves. Severe and prolonged health problems have far-reaching implications on personal finances, family, caregivers, health care professionals, and supportive services. Hence, coping with health conditions has an impact on the individual, the diseases, and the environmental and social contexts of the individual.

Coping with Chronic Health Conditions

Chronic health conditions are associated with the loss of functional ability or diminished well-being. In the absence of a short-term solution to health problems, individuals must find ways to manage and accommodate their physical, cognitive, and affective disabilities, and to manage the environment or context to reduce stress. This process of accommodation can be defined as coping. It is not the scope of this chapter to review the coping literature. It is our intent to identify factors that are pertinent to coping with health conditions in general and with specific diseases in particular.

Ways of Coping

Scharloo et al. (1998) identified these five dimensions within the literature on the structure of illness perception: (a) *identification* refers to the label placed on the disease and its associated symptoms; (b) *causes* refer to how the individual got the disease; (c) *consequences* pertain to the expected outcome of the disease; (d) *timescale* relates to the expectations about the perseverance and characteristics of the illness, and (e) *controllability* refers to the beliefs the individual has about being able to control the disease.

There are numerous definitions and models of coping (e.g., Craig & Edwards, 1983; Folkman & Lazarus, 1980; Thornbury, 1982), but there is no one way to identify the coping process. Pearlin and Schooler (1978) described four functions of coping: prevention of stress from events or situations, alteration of the situation or problem, change in the meaning of the situations, and management of the symptoms or reactions to stress.

Lazarus and Folkman's (1984) cognitive-behavioral theory of stress describes coping as a two-step process that involves appraisal followed by coping. Cognitive coping (also known as primary appraisal) involves the process by which an individual evaluates the degree of threat that is generated by the encounter with the environment. If the stressor is interpreted as positive (e.g., because the stressor is seen as a challenge), positive emotions result. Negative emotions result if the stressor threatens the physical or psychological self, as may occur in the case of chronic health conditions. Secondary appraisal is an assessment of what might and can be done about the situation and whether a given coping strategy will be effective. In this model, coping can be broken down into two general higher order constructs: (a) problem-focused coping or behavioral strategies that aim at managing the external environmental aspects of the stressor and (b) emotion-focused coping or cognitive strategies that regulate the individual's internal state or emotional reactions to the stressor.

Three general coping strategies can be identified. *Problem-focused coping* generally refers to a task orientation in which strategies are used to solve a problem, cognitively reconceptualize it, minimize its effects, or do something to alter the source of the stress. Actions may include such activities as planning, taking direct action, seeking assistance, screening out other activities, and sometimes forcing oneself to wait before acting. These coping styles tend to predominate when an individual feels that something constructive can be done (Maes, Leventhal, & de Ridder, 1996). In contrast, *emotion-focused coping* aims to reduce or manage the emotional distress that is associated with the situation or particular stress. It is associated with a situation or circumstance that must be endured when there is little an individual can do to change the situation (Maes et al.). Examples of this type of coping are crying and anger, self-preoccupation, positive reinterpretation of events, seeking social support, and fantasizing or wishful thinking. *Avoidance coping* is simply avoiding the situation and doing nothing (e.g., Pearlin & Schooler, 1978). When confronted with a stressful situation, the individual may freeze, delay the confrontation, do something else, or deny or suppress awareness of its impact on their life.

Problem-focused coping and cognitive reappraisal are considered more positive strategies than emotion-focused or avoidance coping, as they aim to alter the situation or change the way the stressor is construed. Keller (1988) indicated that problem-solving strategies are used by those capable of controlling their wellness, while emotionally-focused strategies are used effectively by those where the illness is unmanageable. White, Richter, and Fry (1992) found that the use of escape-avoidance and wishful thinking correlated with poor adjustment to diabetes. Roth and Cohen (1986) noted that when a threatening situation is uncontrollable, denial may be the most effective strategy to employ. In our review of the literature, we examined whether cognitive (problem-focused), affective (emotional-focused), and/or physical action are effective to alleviate specific health problems.

Is Age a Risk Factor in Effective Coping?

In our example of Joy in Texas noted earlier, would her coping strategies improve with chronological age as she can use her experiences with various health problems over time? Or would chronological age impede coping effectiveness? The answer, of course, is not simple given the multitude of individual, disease, and social-contextual factors that can affect coping. Aldwin et al. (1996) noted that with age, it is not coping strategies per se that change, but rather management strategies. Older adults tend to use more concrete strategies. They tend to use less interpersonal hostility and escapism. It may be that they have tried these strategies and found them impractical or ineffective. Table 7.1 outlines a summary of findings in which chronological age was found to have a positive, negative, or neutral effect.

Although results summarized in Table 7.1 provide a general picture of the effects of chronological age, it is hypothesized that coping effectiveness may be different for young-old versus old-old (Bennahum, Forman, Vellas, & Albarede, 1997). Young-old individuals, say 65 to 70 years, tend to be in better health and maintain a more viable pool of emotional and family support resources. Their coping is predicted to be more effective when compared to the old-old, say 85 and older, as older individuals tend to have more coexisting chronic conditions, to be more frail and dependent, and to have fewer resources.

Other Individual and Social-Contextual Risk Factors

It is important to note that models of coping emphasize that coping strategy selection is situation specific with some variability accounted for by individual and contextual factors. Though some strategies are deemed to be generally more efficient for specific situations, other strategies may be appropriate for some individuals. For example, some individuals would take active steps toward the remedy of their health problems, while other individuals may resign themselves to their fate.

Three types of illness management strategies have been identified: caring for the disease itself, maintaining a normal lifestyle, and dealing with feelings (Sidell, 1997). The literature has identified three potent individual difference factors (i.e., education, gender, and personality) that can exert a meaningful impact on coping and management of health conditions.

Education

A higher level of education has been found to be a strong positive influence on efficient coping, medication compliance, health problem management, and mastery of technical aids for disability (DeKlerk,

Table 7.1 Summary of Findings Related to Age Differences in Coping with Chronic Health Conditions

Increase in variable with age	Decrease in variable with age	No effect in variable with age
Optimistic and palliative coping strategies in persons with cancer (Halstead & Femsler, 1994)	Emotive strategies in persons with cancer (Halstead & Fermsler, 1994)	Following mastectomy, no differences in active-cognitive (e.g., tried to see positive side) and active-behavioral (e.g., tried to find out more) coping between middle- and old-aged women (Bartmann & Roberto, 1996)
Following mastectomy, 4.5 times as many older than middle-aged women used avoidance coping (e.g., kept my feelings to myself) (Bartmann & Roberto, 1996)	Hostile reaction (McCrae, 1999)	Perseverance (McCrae, 1999)
Isolation of affect (McCrae, 1999)	Rational action (McCrae, 1999)	Seeking help (McCrae, 1999)
Fatalism (McCrae, 1999)	Expression of feelings (McCrae, 1999)	Distraction (McCrae, 1999)
Taking one step at a time (McCrae, 1999)	Positive thinking (McCrae, 1999)	Intellectual denial (McCrae, 1999)
Faith (McCrae, 1999)	Escapist fantasy (McCrae, 1999)	Self-blame (McCrae, 1999)
Distancing (Folkman et al., 1987)	Sedation (McCrae, 1999) (McCrae, 1999)	Social comparison
Acceptance of responsibility (Folkman et al., 1987)	Restraint (McCrae, 1999)	Substitution (McCrae, 1999)
Positive reappraisal (Folkman et al., 1987)	Withdrawal (McCrae, 1999)	Drawing strength from adversity (McCrae, 1999)
Threat minimization (Lerner, 1992)	Self-adaptation (McCrae, 1999)	Avoidance (McCrae, 1999)
	Humor (McCrae, 1999)	Wishful thinking (McCrae, 1999)

(cont.)

Table 7.1 *(Continued)*

Increase in variable with age	Decrease in variable with age	No effect in variable with age
	The total number of coping strategies used (Meeks et al., 1989)	Active forgetting (McCrae, 1999)
	Direct action and social support (Meeks et al., 1989)	Passivity (McCrae, 1999)
	Help-seeking strategies (Meeks et al., 1989)	Indecisiveness (McCrae, 1999)
	Coping through emotional expression (Felton & Revenson, 1987)	Assessing blame (McCrae, 1999)
	Information seeking—but is related to a reduction in the perceived seriousness of illness (Felton & Revenson, 1987)	
	Positive relations (Heidrich & Ryff 1992)	
	Life purpose (Heidrich & Ryff 1992)	
	Interpersonal hostile strategies (Aldwin et al., 1996)	
	Escapism (wishful thinking) (Aldwin et al., 1996)	
	Instrumental action (Aldwin et al., 1996)	
	Social support (Aldwin et al., 1996)	
	Seeking social support (Folkman et al., 1987)	
	Planful problem solving (Folkman et al.,1987)	
	Confrontive (Folkman et al., 1987)	
	Interpersonal aggression (McCrae, 1999)	
	Cognitive reframing (Aldwin et al., 1996)	

Huijsman, & McDonnell, 1997; Verbrugge, Lepkowski, & Konkol, 1991). For example, higher levels of education are associated with increased use of solution-oriented coping strategies, a reduction in the use of resignation, and reduced sympathy-seeking (Krogh et al., 1992). Strain (1996) noted that individuals with a lower level of education are more apt to misunderstand strategies for the treatment of their arthritis. Less education may also restrict communication with health care providers and may delay decision making in response to disease symptoms and treatment options.

Gender

Gender differences also have been shown to exert powerful influences on coping styles. Although gender-related mechanisms in coping have not been thoroughly identified, differences in social roles, support systems, and sources of stress have been noted as important contributors. Folkman and Lazarus (1988) postulated that gender differences in the sources of stress may explain different coping styles between men and women. McCrae (1999) cited a greater use of neurotic coping mechanisms by women (e.g., hostile reaction, expression of feelings, distraction, passivity, wishful thinking, and use of sedation) when coping with stressful situations. In a study of patients with rheumatoid arthritis, Dowdy, Dwyer, Smith, and Wallston (1996) found that women reported more depressive symptoms, negative well-being, passive pain coping, and quality of social support compared to their male counterparts. Folkman, Lazarus, Pimley, and Novacek (1987) noted that men use more self-control (e.g., keeping feelings to oneself) than women, while women use more positive reappraisal than men. Holahan, Moos, Holahan, and Brennan (1995) found that women with cardiac illness used fewer behavioral coping strategies compared to men with similar illness. These findings suggest that gender should be included whenever generalizations about coping with health problems are made.

Personality

Personality has been positively linked with coping with health problems. Neuroticism, locus of control, hardiness, and optimistic outlook all seem to relate to coping efficiency and coping styles. For example, Affleck and Tennen (1992) and Affleck, Urrows, Tennen, and Higgins

(1992) found that neuroticism was related to wishful thinking, catastrophizing, and emotional distress among patients with rheumatoid arthritis. Internal locus of control has been associated with effective coping among patients with arthritis (Brown & Nicassio, 1987) and persons who have hypertension (Powers & Jalowiec, 1987). Hardiness, a characteristic associated with viewing stress as a challenge, and a high level of commitment and sense of control were found in patients who tend to participate in patient education programs and are able to achieve better physiological functioning (Pollock, 1987). Finally, optimists were found to use more active and varied coping strategies than pessimists (Scott, Lindberg, Melin, & Lyttkens, 1994), and pessimists, compared to optimists, had poorer adjustment to illness among individuals with hypertension (Powers & Jalowiec, 1987). In summary, Table 7.2 outlines the effects of individual difference factors in coping with chronic diseases in general. Both positive and negative effects are included.

Social Context

The literature confirms that social context may provide either positive or negative influences on successful coping with health problems. Investigators have particularly focused on the context and constructs of social support and its associated relationship with health (Kriegsman, van Eijk, Penninx, Deeg, & Boeke, 1997; Penninx et al., 1998; Sarason, Sarason, & Pierce, 1990; Sherbourne, Meredith, Rogers, & Ware, 1992). Some findings have demonstrated that social support has a positive effect in reducing morbidity and premature mortality (Belgrave & Lewis, 1994; Felton, 1990; Lanza & Revenson, 1993; Rook & Dooley, 1985; Sugisawa, Liang, & Liu, 1994; Yasuda et al., 1997). In fact, Penninx et al., (1997) reported that moderate to high levels of emotional support reduced the likelihood of dying by half, and it enabled individuals to better cope with a chronic health condition (Sarason et al., 1990; Shreurs & De Ridder, 1997; White et al., 1992) and emotional stress (Berkman et al., 1992; Felton, 1990; Lanza & Revenson, 1993; Penninx et al., 1997). It has also been shown that people with more extensive social networks had higher levels of well-being (Heidrich, 1996) and that subjects who make more upward social comparisons (someone better off than themselves) have higher levels of psychological well-being and lower levels of depression (Heidrich). Those who seek social support have a better functional outcome

Table 7.2 Individual Factors Affecting Coping with Chronic Disease in General

Positive effects

- Higher self-esteem, mastery, and self-efficacy toward "persistence in the face of adversity" were directly associated with less depressive symptoms (Penninx et al., 1998).
- Those who accepted self-management, e.g., no longer sought a cure, scapegoated, or gave up, perceived chronicity positively (Baker & Stern, 1993).
- Those who assented to their illness, embracing the painful reality and reframing, reported the illness as having a diminished "sting" and reconstrued the implications in a positive way (Baker & Stern, 1993).
- People with greater feelings of mastery had a reduced risk of mortality (Penninx et al., 1997a).
- Depressive symptoms were inversely related to religious coping (Koenig et al., 1992).
- Mastery has a positive impact on health related QOL (Kempen et al., 1997b).
- Beliefs in controllability/curability of the disease is related to better functioning (Scharloo et al., 1998).

Negative effects

- Avoidant coping and problem-focused coping predicted greater sickness-related dysfunction (Bombardier et al., 1990).
- More avoidance was associated with greater symptom severity (Bombardier et al., 1990).
- More wishful thinking and self-blame predicted higher levels of depression (Bombardier et al., 1990).
- Anticipatory coping did not diminish psychological disturbance associated with a health downturn (Erdal & Zautra, 1995).
- Accepting responsibility and using more escape-avoidance coping are both associated with more depressive symptoms (Landerville et al., 1994).
- Passive coping is related to worse functioning (Scharloo et al., 1998).
- Considering the illness as a punishment, a strategy, or an enemy resulted in more depressive mood and anxiety (Schussler, 1999).
- Avoidance and acceptance-resignation coping strategies are less effective strategies for life-threatening illness as compared to non-life-threatening illness (Feifel, 1987a).
- Thinking about ways to make a situation better is harmful when it is not accompanied by action (Mattlin et al., 1990).
- Passive-cognitive coping significantly increased reported levels of functional impairment (Lohr et al., 1988).

(Scharloo et al., 1998), increased emotional well-being (Scharloo et al., 1998; Sherbourne et al., 1992), enhanced mobility (Kriegsman et al., 1997), and a better recovery (Wilcox, Kasi, & Berkman, 1994). However, it has also been shown that believing in one's ability to cope without emotional support from others leads to better health outcomes (Wilcox et al., 1994). High levels of instrumental support scores have been associated with increased life satisfaction and reduced symptoms of psychological distress (Revicki & Mitchell, 1990). On the other hand, it should also be noted that some investigators have found that social support can promote negative health outcomes (Antonucci, 1985; Coyne & DeLongis, 1986; Holahan, Moos, Holahan, & Brennan, 1997).

Disease Symptoms, Time Course, and Coping for Life and Nonlife-Threatening Diseases

Basford, Poon, Dowzer, and Booth (chapter 8) examine the effectiveness of different coping strategies for specific diseases. This section summarizes the coping literature on four common themes of disease-related coping: (a) pain, a symptom common to many diseases; (b) depression, a common coexisting condition; (c) changes in coping over the time course of the disease, and (d) differing coping strategies for life-threatening and non-life-threatening health problems.

Pain

Pain is a complex subjective experience incorporating sensory, emotional, and cognitive components, which makes its measurement difficult. The control of pain is an issue for many chronically ill patients but is a particular concern to patients having arthritis or cancer, which tend to strike the middle aged and older adults. Many patients regard pain as an index of disease severity.

A central issue of health coping among older adults is whether they can effectively employ coping strategies that are shown to be efficacious by younger cohorts. Although there is a tremendous amount of individual variation, the learning and memory literature shows that older adults tend to take longer to learn, have lower learning capacity, especially with new information, and tend to be less confident and flexible in the use of learning strategies (Poon, 1985, 2001). Psychological intervention for the control of pain trains patients to take an active independent role in their everyday health. This is contrary to medical therapies in which dependence is encouraged. Commonly utilized coping strategies teach the patient to try to function in spite of the pain, to distract oneself, or to use progressive muscle relaxation. These cognitive coping strategies require continuous effort by the patient in order to be effective. They also require that patients to have confidence in their ability to manage the pain through their own coping strategies and personal resources.

The literature is encouraging in confirming that older adults can effectively use new coping strategies for pain and retain the strategies over a meaningful period of time. In a study with older adults with chronic knee pain, Fry and Wong (1991), found problem-focused coping to be more beneficial than emotion-focused coping. The superiority of problem-focused coping was found to be a result of increased locus of control and competence in pain management. This beneficial effect was still evident 24 weeks later. These investigators also discovered that older adults tended to learn new coping strategies that were consonant with their own coping style. Keefe, Brown, Wallston, and Caldwell (1989) further substantiated the superiority of problem-focused coping, showing that patients with catastrophizing, negative thoughts tend to report higher pain intensities and functional impairments. Keefe and Williams (1990) also found that learned coping-skill training tended to maximize pain reduction in arthritis, compared to arthritis education intervention.

Depression

Depression can be a stand-alone pathology without functional health problems, or it can develop secondarily to diseases. Some chronic health conditions are more strongly associated with depression than others (Penninx et al., 1996). There is also a strong positive relationship between the number of chronic conditions and depressive symptoms (Angel & Angel, 1995; Bazargan, 1996; Burnette & Mui, 1994; Lyness, Duberstein, King, Cox, & Caine, 1999; Palinkas, Wingard, & Barrett Connor, 1990; Roberts, Kaplan, Shema, & Strawbridge, 1997; Vandelisdonk, Furer, Kroonen, & Marijnissen, 1992). Penninx et al. (1996) reported that individuals with three or more chronic health conditions scored twice as high on depression as those with no chronic conditions. Depression is therefore a major confounding factor in the treatment of chronic diseases and functional impairments.

Lewinsohn, Hoberman, Teri, and Hautzinger (1985) developed a model relating depression and functional impairment among older adults, as follows:

1. Physical disease increases the likelihood and subsequent onset of depression in older persons only when it is associated with functional impairment.
2. Functional impairment, whether associated with a particular chronic health condition or not, increases the probability of subsequent depression.
3. The greater the degree of functional impairment, the greater the risk of onset of depression.
4. Depression can predispose an older individual to develop illness or exacerbate an existing one.
5. Depression can result in functional impairment at a greater level than is physically indicated by the severity of the disease, resulting in an excess disability.

Patients who are depressed tend to use different and less efficient strategies in coping compared to patients who are not. Specifically, patients who are depressed tend to use more avoidance-coping and emotion-focused coping compared to more active cognitive and behavioral coping among those who are not depressed (Kalfoss, 1993; Rosenberg, Peterson, & Hayes, 1987). Active coping has been reported to be the strongest predictor of changing mental health over time. The subjects who were depressed who could use active coping showed more improvements over time compared to those who did not use active coping (Sherbourne, Hays, & Wells, 1995). These findings indicate that depression is associated with learned helplessness and perceived control, which in turn tend to dictate the coping strategies employed by an individual.

A controversial question is whether depression increases the difficulty of older adults in learning new information, such as new coping strategies. This issue is controversial because there are findings to support that it does (e.g., Hart & Kwentus, 1987; La Rue, D'Elia, Clark, Spar, & Jarvik, 1986; Sweeney, Wetzler, Stokes, & Kocsis, 1989) and that it does not (e.g., Miller & Lewis, 1977; Niederehe, 1986; Popkin, Gallagher, Thompson, & Moore, 1982; Vitiello, Prinz, Poon, & Williams, 1990). In a meta-analysis of the data, Poon (1992) concluded that depression by itself is not a sufficient condition to degrade learning and memory; however, if early dementia is a coexisting condition, then learning and memory are definitely compromised.

Coping Over the Time Course of the Disease

Much of the research on coping over the time course of a disease involved middle-aged and older adults. Signs, symptoms, and severity of any disease change over time. Coping and coping strategies change over time as well. Morse and Johnson (1991) developed the Illness Constellation Model that defines four stages of the illness experience, beginning with the *stage of uncertainty*. This stage occurs when the individual detects or suspects signs of illness, endeavoring to make sense of the symptoms by finding a meaning and level of severity. Stage two is the *stage of disruption*, which begins when the individual chooses to seek medical help, or a medical diagnosis is confirmed. The third stage is *striving to regain the self*, in which the person attempts to make sense of what happened while attempting to predict future ramifications of the disease. Stage four, *regaining wellness*, occurs when the individual begins to assert order to reclaim control through questioning treatment, seeking information about diagnosis, getting test results, and determining the outlook.

Large intra- and inter-individual differences in cognitive strategies are often found at the beginning of the disease as individuals pass through different moods, evaluation, and coping. Kruse (1987) indicated that denial was the foremost reaction with cancer and stroke patients when the diagnosis was first made. With the passage of time, cancer patients tend to show severe depression, indicating that they are aware of the seriousness of the disease. Stroke patients, on the other hand, tend to be less inclined to show depressive symptoms, often focusing on how to avoid becoming aware of their illness. Over the course of chronic diseases, coping strategies change with the functions of time, severity, and the effectiveness of specific strategies. New coping strategies may also be incorporated. Alternatively, coping skills may be reduced, resulting from feelings of being overwhelmed by the burden of disease. Revenson and Felton (1989) found that increasing disability in rheumatoid arthritis over a 6-month period was associated with less acceptance of the illness and more wishful thinking. The literature shows that coping over the course of a disease is a dynamic process, depending on treatment progress, the effectiveness of coping at a specific time, and the involvement of pain and disabilities.

Coping for Life and Nonlife-Threatening Health Problems

When an individual realizes that the course of a disease is not life-threatening and could improve over time, they often employ problem-focused coping strategies (Lazarus & Folkman, 1984). However, when a life-threatening or hopeless condition is detected, they use more emotion-focused coping strategies. Hopelessness increases with impending death in cancer patients, reflecting the fact that they no longer adhere to false hopes but possess a realistic attitude and an acceptance of death (Lerner, 1992).

From this perspective, resignation is a positive coping strategy. Alternatively, when the disease is not terminal, hopelessness has a negative effect and can lead to exacerbation of the disease.

Five different processes of coping with dying and death have been identified (Kruse, 1987) as cited below:

1. The acceptance of dying and death and the search for possibilities that life still has to offer.
2. An increase in resignation and bitterness. During this phase, life is viewed as a burden with the finite nature of existence being felt.
3. The fact that the individual is still performing meaningful functions results in the feeling of a new sense of life as the fear of death eases.
4. The prevention of existential threat from being the sole focus of experience.
5. The individual comes to terms with death after going through a deep depression.

Summary of Coping Strategies Associated with Chronic Diseases

Our review has summarized the literature on ways of coping with chronic diseases and their concomitant individual, contextual, and disease-related impacts on older adults. The coping literature has grown exponentially from the mid-1960s to the present. Coyne and Racioppo (2000) estimated that there are close to 23,000 published papers on coping. Our literature search on coping strategies dealing with coexisting chronic diseases, aging, and the aged netted few entries even though our search encompassed 12 databases, which selected 7,139 papers using our keywords. From these, we selected 483 of the most promising studies to review. The results of our review of the literature on coping strategies and chronic illnesses of older adults, according to the 12 diseases selected, are presented by Basford et al. in chapter 8 (see Sample Review Model and Review Synthesis Sections). On the basis of reported data in the literature, we summarized the coping strategies for the 12 diseases according to their (a) being effective and regularly used, (b) being ineffective or infrequently used, or (c) needing further research or resulting in no indication of the strategy's effectiveness.

Our summary of coping strategies for chronic health conditions is presented in Table 7.3, according to these categories: (a) cognitive,

Table 7.3 Coping Strategies Used by Older Adults with Chronic Health Conditions

Coping strategy	Recommended or frequently used +	Need further research. No indication of effectiveness 0	Not recommended or not used often −
Cognitive:			
Self-criticism			Viney & West-brook, 1986
			Koenig et al., 1988; Landerville et al., 1994
Avoidant coping		Bombardier et al., 1990	
• Went on as if nothing had happened			
• Avoided the situation			
Cognitive restructuring	Felton & Revenson, 1987; Kalfoss, 1993; Landerville et al., 1994; Manne & Zautra, 1990		Kalfoss, 1993*; Koenig et al., 1988
• Rediscovered what was important in life			
• Changed something about myself			
• Got away from it for a while/went on holiday			
• Reminded myself of how much worse things could be			
• Thought about how a person I admired would handle it and used that as a model			
Time heals all wounds	Koenig et al., 1988		
Looked at problems objectively	Kalfoss, 1993		
• Tried to analyze the problem to understand it better			
Learning through experience	Kalfoss, 1993		
• Came out of the experience better than I came in			
Positive reinterpretation	Agrawal & Pandey, 1998		

(cont.)

Table 7.3 (Continued)

Coping strategy	Recommended or frequently used	Need further research. No indication of effectiveness	Not recommended or not used often
Autonomy			
• Try to maintain autonomy	De Ridder et al., 1997		
• I myself would like to decide how I spend my days			
Experience of prior hardships			
Carried on as usual	Kalfoss, 1993		Koenig et al., 1988
• Waited to see what happened before doing anything			Koenig et al., 1988
Confrontive coping	Feifel et al., 1987; Landerville et al., 1994; Kalfoss, 1993; Michael, 1996		
• Knew what had to be done, so doubled my efforts to make things work			
• Confronted loss			
Self-controlling	Do Rozario, 1997; Landerville et al., 1994		
• I have empowerment and choice			
Accepting responsibility			Landerville et al., 1994
Planful problem-solving	Landerville et al., 1994		
Optimism	Kalfoss, 1993		
Positive attitude	Clark et al., 1996; Koenig et al., 1988		

Table 7.3 (*Continued*)

Coping strategy	Recommended or frequently used	Need further research. No indication of effectiveness	Not recommended or not used often
Meaningful engagement in life			
• Participation and interest	Do Rozario, 1997		
Cognitive			
• Positive thinking			
• Tried to see things from the other person's point of view			
• Bargained or compromised to get something positive from the situation	De Ridder et al., 1997; Eakes, 1993; Heidrich & Ryff, 1992; Kalfoss, 1993; Michael, 1996		
• Gained control over life direction			
Cognitive optimizing			
• Compared themselves favorably with others			
• Looked at those who are worse off	Baker & Stern, 1993	Johnson & Barber, 1999	Koenig et al., 1988
• Realized others in same situation or worse			
Distancing	Landerville et al., 1994		
Mental disengagement	Agrawal & Pandey, 1998		
Compare to someone living effectively with illness	Baker & Stern, 1993		
Selective withdrawal		Johnson & Barber, 1999	
Living a story of "life as normal"			
• Try to make it part of everyday life and keep things in perspective, changing the story as it is enacted (reframing)	Robinson, 1993		

(cont.)

Table 7.3 (*Continued*)

Coping strategy	Recommended or frequently used	Need further research. No indication of effectiveness	Not recommended or not used often
Self-management			
• Cognitive system management	Lorig et al., 1999		
• Enhance communication with doctor			
Accept it	Agrawal & Pandey, 1998; Koenig et al., 1988		
Talk to others	Clark et al., 1996		
Read		Raleigh, 1992	
Problem-focused			
• Made a plan of action and followed it	Bombardier et al., 1990; Kalfoss, 1993; Michael, 1996		
• Implemented changes	Agrawal & Pandey, 1998		
Active coping			
Help from professional	Koenig et al., 1988		
Seek/receive help from others	Norburn et al., 1995		
Planning/preparing beforehand	Koenig et al., 1988; Norburn et al., 1995; Agrawal & Pandey, 1998		
• Plan shopping trip			
• Stocking up when going to the store			
Lowered expectations			Koenig et al., 1988
Take one at a time	Koenig et al., 1988		

Table 7.3 (*Continued*)

Coping strategy	Recommended or frequently used	Need further research. No indication of effectiveness	Not recommended or not used often
Maintaining sociability		Johnson & Barber, 1999	
Imagery	Hasitavej, 1995		
Self-blame			Bombardier et al., 1990; Felton & Revenson, 1987; Kalfoss, 1993; Manne & Zautra, 1990
• Brought problem on myself (Bombardier et al., 1990			
• Criticized myself (Kalfoss, 1993			
Affective:			
Express Emotions	Kalfoss, 1993; Michael, 1996; De Ridder et al., 1997	Raleigh, 1992; Eakes, 1993; Felton & Revenson, 1987	Heidrich & Ryff, 1992; Kalfoss, 1993; Koenig et al., 1988
• Crying or cursing			
• Draw on past experiences			
• Daydreamed of a better place than the one I was in			
• Avoided being with people			
• Took it out on other people			
• Fluctuated emotions			
Helplessness			Viney & Westbrook, 1986
Denial	De Ridder et al., 1997		Agrawal & Pandey, 1998
Resignation	De Ridder et al., 1997		

(*cont.*)

Table 7.3 *(Continued)*

Coping strategy	Recommended or frequently used	Need further research. No indication of effectiveness	Not recommended or not used often
Cognitive and affective: Praying/hoping/spirituality	Clark et al., 1996; Do Rozario, 1997; Koenig et al., 1988; Koenig et al., 1992; Lehr & Kruse, 1992; Raleigh, 1992; Roberson, 1992		
Wishful thinking • Hoped for a miracle		Bombardier et al., 1990	Manne & Zautra, 1990
Wish-fulfilling fantasy • Wished the situation would go away • Wished I could change what has happened		(Felton & Revenson, 1987	Kalfoss, 1993
Maintained my pride/kept a stiff upper lip			
Accepted it	Lehr & Kruse, 1992		Kalfoss, 1993
Information seeking • Asked relative or friend for advice	Felton & Revenson, 1987; Kalfoss, 1993; Koenig et al.,		Kalfoss, 1993

Table 7.3 (Continued)

Coping strategy	Recommended or frequently used	Need further research. No indication of effectiveness	Not recommended or not used often
Fatalism	1988; Roberson, 1992		
• You have only yourself to blame			
• Disease just happens to you	De Ridder et al., 1997		
Threat minimization	Felton & Revenson, 1987		Kalfoss, 1993
• Tried to forget the whole thing			
• Tried to keep feelings to myself			
• Went on as if nothing was happening			
• Kept others from knowing how bad things were			
Avoid interpersonal conflicts	Clark et al., 1996		
Empowerment	McDermott, 1995		Koenig et al., 1988
Carried on for others' sake			
Alternate channels to human friendship	Clark et al., 1996		
• Pet, teddy bear, book			
Seeking social support	Agrawal & Pandey, 1998; Bombardier et al., 1990; Carruth & Boss, 1990; Clark et al., 1996; De		

(cont.)

Table 7.3 *(Continued)*

Coping strategy	Recommended or frequently used	Need further research. No indication of effectiveness	Not recommended or not used often
	Ridder et al., 1997; Do Rozario, 1997; Koenig et al., 1988; Laferriere & Hamel Bissell, 1994; Landerville et al., 1994; Lehr & Kruse, 1992; Roberts et al., 1995; Rybarczyk et al., 1999		
Cognitive and physical: Get busy	Clark et al., 1996; Koenig et al., 1988; Raleigh, 1992		
Limited activities • Do things less often/more slowly • Avoid lifting heavy objects	Koenig et al., 1988; Norburn et al., 1995		

Table 7.3 (*Continued*)

Coping strategy	Recommended or frequently used	Need further research. No indication of effectiveness	Not recommended or not used often
Self-management			
• Stretching, exercise, strengthening	Hasitavej, 1995; Heidrich & Ryff, 1992; Lorig et al., 1999		
• Diet, exercise	Koenig et al., 1988		
Helped others more needy	Folden, 1990; Norburn et al., 1995)		
Change living surroundings		Johnson & Barber, 1999	
Alcohol, tranquilizers			Koenig et al., 1988
Seek medical assistance	Clark et al., 1996		
Folk remedies	Montbriand & Laing, 1991; Roberson 1992		
Exercise	Butler et al., 1998; Hickey et al., 1995; Koenig et al., 1988; Morey et al., 1989; Shin, 1999; Stewart et al., 1994		
Stretching	Valentine-Garzon, 1992		

(*cont.*)

Table 7.3 (*Continued*)

Coping strategy	Recommended or frequently used	Need further research. No indication of effectiveness	Not recommended or not used often
Stress reduction	Hasitavej, 1995; Roberson, 1992		
Comply with general health knowledge	Clark et al., 1996		
Education	Ostwald et al., 1990		
Reminiscence therapy	Smith & Couch, 1990		
Staying active	Laferriere & Hamel Bissell, 1994		
Rehabilitation therapy	Rijken & Dekker, 1998		
Use situational therapy contextual cues	Clark et al., 1996		
• Wait for nice day before going out			
Assistive devices	Norbum et al., 1995	Johnson & Barber, 1999	
Dependence	De Ridder et al., 1997		
Cognitive, affective, and physical:			
Get involved in social activity	Clark et al., 1996;		
• Join club	Koenig et al., 1988		
Action	Heidrich & Ryff, 1992; Kalfoss, 1993		
• Inspired to do something creative			

(b) affective, (c) cognitive and affective, (d) cognitive and physical, and (e) cognitive, affective, and physical. Further, these strategies are classified as (a) recommended or frequently used, (b) need further research or no indication of effectiveness, and (c) not recommended or not often used. In this manner, the reader can select evidence-based coping methods that have been shown to be efficacious for specific situations.

The Fruits of Our Literature Search

Four general conclusions that may contribute to an understanding of this phenomenon can be drawn from the results of our quest for answers on coping with comorbidity among older adults. First, the coping and health coping literature is extensive as exhibited by its exponential growth in the last 30 years. Second, extensive literature is available to inform researchers and clinicians about the effectiveness of specific coping strategies for selected specific situations and diseases. These strategies are summarized in this and the following two chapters. Third, we were unable to uncover literature that could provide answers to our questions about evaluating the impact of, and coping with, coexisting chronic diseases. The extant studies on health coping either examine coping with a specific disease or health condition, or control for the confounding of other existing diseases or conditions. Fourth, because comorbidity is common among older adults and has significant medical and psychological implications for the quality of their everyday lives, a new generation of research is needed to test and extend currently available models of coping strategies for dealing with multiple chronic conditions.

Nonetheless, how do we use our extant knowledge toward better understanding of the basic mechanisms of health coping and evidence-based intervention now? The signs that guide us from here to there are many and often controversial. The last section of this chapter addresses this question from three perspectives: We examine the most current reviews of the stress and coping literature regarding strengths and weaknesses; we summarize suggested new directions from these reviews; and we share our thoughts on needed directions in research on health coping in general and coping for comorbidity in particular.

Self-Criticism Among Stress and Coping Researchers

Introspection among stress and coping researchers tends to be harsh in terms of how they view their previous accomplishments in this area of research (Lazarus, 2000; Somerfield & McCrea, 2000). For example, Somerfield and McCrae noted that "coping is among the most widely studied topics in contemporary psychology. However, the explosion of interest in coping has yielded little and the field is in crisis" (p. 620). In their examination of current research on coping and its application, Somerfield and McCrae indicated that the numerous findings from this field have been criticized for being disappointing, tentative, modest, sterile, stagnated, and trivial. A series of integrated papers on the topic in 2000, published in the *American Psychologist* (Coyne & Racioppo, 2000; Cramer, 2000; Lazarus, 2000; Somerfield & McCrea, 2000; Tennen, Affleck, Armeli, & Carney, 2000), collectively noted serious problems in conceptual and methodological issues, research designs, the neglect of unconscious reactions to stress, the narrow selection of adaptational outcomes, and a clear understanding of the relationship between coping mechanisms and clinical applications. These criticisms made us more sensitive during our examination of the construct of successful and effective coping with multiple chronic illnesses among older adults, the means of measuring coping, current models of coping, pertinent mechanisms not previously considered, and for those in clinical intervention, the applicability of known successful kinds of intervention. These reviews clearly signal the need for the next generation of research.

Strengths and Weaknesses in Stress and Coping Studies

In spite of the harsh criticisms levied at the collective research in the field of stress and coping, certain studies have produced important findings and theoretical models. Pioneers in the field (Folkman & Lazarus, 1980; Moos, 1976; Pearlin & Schooler, 1978) have made significant theoretical and methodological contributions to address the critical question of human survival, namely, how to recognize, conceptualize, and measure illness-related stress and alleviate it. Indeed, much research has shown that clear and positive intervention results in behavioral medicine in pain and stress management, depression, medication compliance, illness adjustment, and so on (e.g., Davidson, Williams, Nezami, Bice & DeQuattro, 1991; Fry & Wong, 1991; Roter et al., 1998). These pioneers and others have continued to create new directions in the field (e.g., Folkman & Moskowitz, 2000; Lazarus, 1999). In our opinion, the harsh criticisms have reflected frustration with the field's inability to break out of the methodological doldrums, in which some researchers tend to perpetuate existing flaws in design and methodology without thinking through their substantive research questions. The criticisms: (a) the use of cross-sectional designs to make conclusions about within-subject changes, and (b) the use of incomplete randomized samples or the lack of adequate controls in making sweeping conclusions on the specific processes or effectiveness of specific intervention point to the need for multiple studies and multiple methods in pursuing the research questions.

In terms of health coping, measurable physical symptoms (such as pain and physical disabilities), affect (such as frustration, apprehension, anxiety, worry, and depression), and relative changes in signs and symptoms are real to the patient in the course of the health problems. However, given the same constellation of symptoms, perceptions of the severity and impact may be different for different individuals. There is no argument from coping researchers that health coping is disease-, context-, and individual-specific. Coyne and Racioppo (2000) admonished that these interactions, although recognized as critical, are not addressed adequately in the literature. The symptom checklist methodology, which has generated a good portion of the coping research, is too general and simplistic. Different individuals in different situations with the same symptoms vary greatly in their coping and their perceived outcome. Coyne and Racioppo went so far as to issue this warning in bold type: **"Warning! Hundreds of studies have established that use of this instrument is unlikely to yield findings of substantive importance and that the risk of confounded and otherwise spurious results is high"** (p. 659). Not all researchers, however, share the severity of their criticism (Lazarus, 2000).

It is clear that the thrust of the criticism stating that the research so far has been disappointing ia aimed at our inability to understand clearly and delineate the roles, interactions, and potential confounding among specific stress, context, and individual interaction in coping over time. This may be particularly true for health coping research, where individual differences can be very pronounced in signs and symptoms. Even within the same class of chronic conditions, severity could alter symptoms and perception, and differences in personality and coping styles could further exacerbate differences in perception. Individual differences in their support systems could also further complicate the picture. To treat a number of individuals with the same health condition as a homogeneous group might produce large within-group variability to the point that it may be as large or larger than between-group variability. For these reasons, we can excuse researchers for not tackling the thorny issue of coping with more than one health condition. However, the resolution of this methodological shortcoming can now be achieved using multiple designs and methods.

Suggested Solutions to Coping Research Issues

Based on the criticisms just alluded to, the constellation of constructive solutions range from "razing the slum before building further"—to re-conceptualizing more practical expectations of what coping alone can do toward adaptation—to admonishing researchers—to reviewing basic research principles prior to designing studies in coping. However, should generic symptom checklists that are commonly employed in stress and coping research be summarily abolished (Coyne & Racioppo, 2000)? The answer, of course, is dependent on the research question: Any conveniently available instrument should not be used without sufficient assurance of construct and predictive validity and reliability that would provide a meaningful answer to the research question. The criticism is deserved that too many researchers tend to use instruments that are universally employed without considering the suitability to their particular research questions. The criticism is also warranted that some researchers are lax (or not sufficiently informed) in establishing the psychometric relevance of their instruments prior to application.

Another suggestion is that coping strategies alone are not end-all solutions for successful adaptation, and researchers and clinicians should moderate their expectations of the amount of variance in coping strategies that could account for the outcome measures (Pearlin, 1991; Somerfield & McCrae, 2000). This suggestion is predicated on individual differences in the perception of stress, personality, and coping styles that may or may not be situation specific, as well as on the social and context support available to that individual. From this perspective, clinicians should also be aware that not all coping methods work for every person and that some persons are more amenable than others to the use of coping strategies.

Although disease, context, and individual interactions are deemed important for understanding health coping mechanisms, and therefore successful adaptation, the question arises as to whether understanding these interactions is as important as it has been touted to be (Lazarus, 2000). This is both a theoretical and empirical question. From a theoretical perspective, coping, by definition, is individual and context-dependent, so any examination of successful coping without considering these factors would be flawed. Some coping processes may be universal or situation- or time-specific, and therefore may depend less on the characteristics of the individual or other concomitant factors. These interactions, or lack thereof, can be tested empirically. From a practical perspective, only a few "mega" studies can vary or control *all* relevant variables; thus, smaller sequential studies may be needed to understand relevant mechanisms. Nevertheless, consideration of these interactions is central to the next generation of research on coping and health coping.

And what may some of these next steps be to expand our extant knowledge? As noted earlier, more thoughtful consideration in basic research principles would eliminate the use of nonvalidated instruments and the attempts to answer longitudinal questions using cross-sectional design, and would increase specificity in the selection of both independent and dependent variables. As the pendulum of scientific investigation swings, current discontent with generalized coping research has facilitated descriptive, longitudinal studies on specific types of coping that focus on small samples or even individual-level studies that have limited generalizability (e.g., Tennen et al., 2000). Instead of searching for global models, some researchers go back to basics to attempt to understand coping at the microanalysis level. Here the focus is on the individual level. As noted by Lazarus (2000), this type of research focuses on "cognitive-motivational-relational centered mediation (e.g., appraising), a longitudinal (or prospective) research style, and an effort to obtain microanalytic data in a framework that is process centered and holistic" (p. 668). Other research seeks to examine relevant coping mechanisms that previously have not been the focus, such as unconscious psychological processes (Cramer, 2000), positive as well as negative effects in coping (Folkman & Moskowitz, 2000), and exceptionally long-lived individuals who qualify as "expert survivors" (Martin et al., 1992).

Conclusions

The challenges are set for gerontologists and health care professionals to provide older adults with practical solutions to their problem of living with multiple health problems. One challenge is that this problem is pervasive and awaits everyday solutions. Another is that the extant literature has clearly delineated and posed the methodological and theoretical problems for the next generation of research. From the methodological perspective, we found that too many studies were one-shot attempts to examine complex phenomena. We believe it is important instead to use multiple methods and programmatic approaches with built-in replications. Owing to the large intra- and intersubject variability among older adults, sampling must be done with care, or findings may not replicate.

We have begun qualitative studies in which older adults in focus groups have told us in their own words what strategies they have used to cope with comorbidity day to day (see Penrod et al. in chapter 9). We believe this was a start in order to sort out the independent and dependent variables. However, we would like to find out what the similarities and differences are between their doctor's medical diagnoses of their comorbidities and the older person's own perceptions. We would also like to know whether these assessments make a difference in the older adults' ways of coping and their effectiveness. How do older people define successful coping? How do people cope when they experience more than one chronic condition at a time? Are there different methods of coping for primary and tertiary conditions? How do they make these decisions? Do different types of people use different coping styles? We would like to see the variability of disease impacts and consistency of coping over time. Are there limited sets of coping strategies available to a particular individual? How often do they use specific strategies? Under what conditions do they learn new strategies? As noted earlier, we began with several focus groups (see chapter 9); we are now following the coping behaviors of individuals in those groups according to their own descriptions in their daily logs. We plan to select new samples to test our new hypotheses over time. It will be an exciting journey.

Chapter 8

Coping with Specific Chronic Health Conditions

Lynn Basford, Leonard W. Poon, Clare Dowzer, and Andrew Booth

I n the previous chapter we explore the paradigms of coping with comorbidity among older adults as explained within the extant literature. On examination of this literature, from quite diverse sources, it became obvious that it failed to define how individuals cope with multiple chronic conditions. Confronted with this rather surprising result, the review team used an agreed-upon model that would enable examination of the literature in order to provide information on coping within a specific disease entity. The rationale for our model was based on the assumption that the scientific community would have explored how older adults who are faced with chronic illness associated with a particular disease would, through necessity, have used health coping behaviors.

Our main task was to extrapolate the evidence of these behaviors with a view towards gaining an understanding of coping strategies that are used with different chronic conditions manifested by a particular disease. In doing so, we continued to apply the same rigorous process used in stage one that could extract information from both the qualitative and quantitative scientific literature. We believed this would produce a rich source of information and evidence of coping strategies that have been used by older adults with a single chronic illness, and would therefore offer insights into the relationship that some of these chronic disease entities have, by nature, with other clinical conditions (comorbidity). This relationship, we hypothesized, would be more evident as the disease reached a terminal or tertiary point. For example, it is widely known that chronic cardiac insufficiency has a direct causal affect on other major systems of the body, in particular the respiratory and renal systems. Each system failure could be classified as a prime chronic disease in its own right. This is particularly so if the symptoms require medical intervention or indeed a coping strategy that supersedes coping with other symptoms that are presented with other disease states as a matter of priority (perceived or actual).

The review team also felt that some disease classifications were in themselves a comorbid entity affecting specific body systems at different points along the disease trajectory. Diabetes mellitus and cancer are classic examples. Though our focus was to determine the paradigms of older adults' coping with chronic illnesses from a symptomatic approach, we were mindful that living with such health conditions may also have a direct effect on the mental of the individual as well as the physical health concerned. For example, depression is often observed in the clinical situation when an older person has one or more chronic illnesses. This condition could be associated with a person's loss of positive body image and physical capabilities, reduced power and status in the family unit, feelings of impending doom about their own demise, or with the effects of a chemical imbalance or hormonal imbalance on brain cells. Several authors have identified the correlation between depression and any chronic health condition (Broe et al., 1998; Freedland et al., 1991; Grady, Maisog, Horwitz, & Ungerleider, 1994; Koenig, 1998; Steffens et al., 1999).

Given these multiple variables, it is clear that defining comorbidity is a multifactorial concept and cannot be considered from the sole perspective of a pathophysiological dimension. Other influences related to the physical might include psychological, environmental, sociological, and spiritual aspects of health, which may pervade chronic health problems experienced by older people. Such concepts require a holistic understanding of human functioning that recognizes the intricate nature and complicated dimensions of health, thereby enabling the older person to maintain and restore health, even to prevent illness, by using a range of effective coping mechanisms.

The application of holistic paradigms in medical practice is a relatively recent phenomenon, because modern medicine has been co-

cooned in the scientific model, which has reduced health and illness to their infinite component parts (i.e., a reductionistic model). Although there are perceived advantages to this form of microscopic interpretation and classification of disease pathways and entities, it does negate a comprehensive understanding of secondary interrelated diseases or the malfunctioning of the body associated with a chronic illness. Further, the scientific or clinical approach has served to foster medical diagnosis and treatment from a specialist perspective that maintains the distinction of viewing chronic illness in older people as a single disease entity. This singular view of illness may be one of the reasons the literature has not addressed comorbid issues in a meaningful or comprehensive manner, which forced our review team to explore other avenues to explain the complex issues and relationships of disease entities and the ways in which older people effectively cope with multiple chronic health conditions. To overcome this conceptual conundrum, we relied on a process of deduction to identify how comorbidity is partially the result of a common pathological process or the complications of the natural course of the disease by which one bodily system affects another. For example, Kaplan and Feinstein (1974) illustrate the interrelationship of diabetes mellitus, cardiovascular disease, chronic obstructive pulmonary disease, and heart failure.

Refining Disease Categories for Review of Coping Strategies

The financial and time limitations on our search required that we judge which particular diseases to focus on, based on their effects with regard to (a) the higher incidence of mortality and morbidity, (b) the burden of disease on the individual, (c) the effects on the caregiver and society, (d) the economic costs, and (e) the overall reduction in quality of life. We acknowledged that some diseases are classified under an all-inclusive generic umbrella. For instance, the term "cancer" does not just represent a single disease in and of itself, but applies to a whole range of disease entities that are associated with a common physiological manifestation of abnormal cell reproduction; Falvo (1991) identified 100 different types of cancers or neoplastic diseases. Obviously, our project could not do justice to this one disease classification since it has a range of 100 subsets. Therefore, we limited our review of the literature on comorbidity to the four most common types of cancer among the older population, based on their incidence rates, the need to deploy coping strategies (particularly with radical invasive therapies), and gender-specific cancers that can cause changes in body image or behavior, such as breast or prostate cancer. From this list of chronic conditions, we made further selections to include a range of disabilities (e.g., mobility, vision, psychological distress, difficulty in breathing, etc.) and to prevent our classification from being dominated by cancer-related disorders. For instance, chronic health problems that require a profound change in behavior were included, based on the need for coping with the behavioral change.

We narrowed the list to 12 diseases, according to the following basic criteria: (a) they were the chief causes of chronic illness in older people, (b) they caused loss of functioning due to disability in older adults, and (c) they impinged on their quality of life and ability to maintain their independence. In addition, we included two kinds of cancers associated with gender. The 12 diseases in the final list were cardiovascular disease, stroke and hypertension, respiratory disease, diabetes mellitus, arthritis, lung cancer, colorectal cancer, prostatic cancer, breast cancer, osteoporosis/fractures, visual impairments, and hearing impairments. The rationale for including these diseases also entailed a discussion and judgment of whether the strategies for coping with the disease had cognitive, affective, or physical effects. In addition, the team demonstrated a certain degree of arbitrary decision-making, given the necessity to lump otherwise discrete disease entities under a generic classification such as cardiovascular disease.

Continuing to use a rigorous systematic approach, we analyzed each disease entity, using the following categories:

- incidence and prevalence
- the most common morbidities
- disease pattern and prognosis
- disease influences on functioning from cognitive, affective, and physical perspectives
- coping strategies used to embrace these three areas of functioning.
- individual variances when engaged in coping strategies
- the relationship or value of social support or social structures to aid effective coping

To illustrate this model, we present the full findings on cardiovascular disease below. Because of the confines of this chapter, we offer only a synthesis of the coping strategies for the other 11 disease classifications in a later section. (A full breakdown can be seen in our final project report.)

Sample Review Model: Coping Strategies Used With Cardiovascular Disease

Incidence and Prevalence

Twenty-one million cases of heart disease were reported in the United States in 1995 (National Vital Health and Statistics Report [NVHSR], 1999). Heart disease is the leading cause of death for older Americans, accounting for 481,458 deaths in 1994 (world Health Organization [WHO] 1999) and 726,974 deaths in 1997 (NVHSR). Heart disease was also the leading cause of death in Europe for 1998 (WHO). Hypertension accounted for 13,534 deaths in 1997, with the majority of these being older individuals. Sixty-four percent of males and more than three-quarters of women aged 75 and older have hypertension (NVHSR).

Most Common Comorbidities

Steffens et al. (1999) reported that 8% of coronary heart disease patients met the criteria for major depression. Among patients with congestive heart failure, major depression was identified in 37% compared to 26% in cardiac patients without congestive heart failure. Koenig (1998) reported that patients with congestive heart failure were more likely suffer from a myocardial infarction, hypertension, respiratory disorders, and diabetes than patients with heart failure of a noncongestive type. Twenty-six percent of hypertensive patients were reported to have a concomitant diagnosis of coronary heart disease, congestive heart failure, or stroke, respectively (Gambassi et al., 1998). The most frequent co-occurring chronic conditions associated with heart disease among a women's health and aging study (Fried, BandeenRoche, Kaser, & Guralnik, 1999) were visual impairment, arthritis, or hypertension. These were ranked fourth, sixth, and seventh, respectively, with proportions of the population having both diseases: 17%, 14%, and 13%, respectively.

Disease Pattern and Prognosis

As humans age, the coronary arteries that supply blood to the heart muscle become progressively narrower (arteriosclerosis), resulting from the formation of a fatty plaque. This narrowing of the arteries is known as coronary heart disease. Hypertension places a great strain on the arteries and over time they become scarred and inelastic. Eventually this can lead to atherosclerosis, stroke, or a myocardial infarction. Congestive heart failure is brought about when the heart muscle becomes too weak to maintain an adequate cardiac output to meet the body's demands for oxygen. This usually results from the heart's being either overworked or damaged, often as a result of hypertension, atherosclerosis, or a myocardial infarction.

Cardiovascular Disease Influences on Functioning

Cognitive

Cardiac insufficiency will result in a reduced blood volume and thus a decreased cerebral blood supply. Hypoxia resulting from cardiac insufficiency may reduce cognitive impairment.

Affective

The unpredictable nature of cardiovascular disease and the associated fear of having a heart attack or the fear of impending death may cause an increase in emotional state.

Physical

The impact of cardiovascular disease on the physical system depends on the severity of the disease. Treatment for cardiovascular disease advocates exercise for the control and prevention of further complications. However, if an attack is severe enough, cardiovascular disease may result in disability from fatigue, weakness, activity intolerance, and shortness of breath.

Coping Strategies With Cardiovascular Disease

As stated earlier, our model identified coping strategies that are used within a cognitive, physical, or affective frame of reference, but not all coping strategies were clearly identified with one distinct category. Some were based on either cognitive and affective, or cognitive and physical, or all three. For the most part, it became obvious that for anyone to use effective coping strategies with cardiovascular disease, a degree of cognition was necessary. There were exceptions to this rule, as the use of assistive devices or technical aides employed both the physical and the affective domain. Key coping activities used by persons with cardiovascular disease are as follows:

Cognitive

Coping strategies included confrontive behavior (Feifel, 1987); searching for a meaning either from the perspective of acceptance or unfound or found meaning and optimistic behavior (King, Rowe, Kimble, & Zerwick, 1998); medication knowledge (Powers & Jalowiec, 1987); solution-orientation such as information seeking, handling problems in stages; trying out new solutions (Krogh et al., 1992); setting goals; making use of past experiences; trying to change the situation and discussing the problem objectively (Krogh et al., 1992); and having insight about and knowledge of the disease (Powers & Jalowiec, 1998).

Affective

Coping strategies that fell under the affective domain included descriptions of resignation, such as hopelessness, fate, acceptance of the situation, praying, doing nothing, withdrawing, daydreaming, not worrying; or descriptors for an emotional response, for example, getting mad, being nervous, taking it out on others, worrying, wanting to be alone, expecting the worst, blaming others, and crying (Krogh et al., 1992).

Cognitive and Affective

Examples of coping strategies used under this category were: avoidance (King et al., 1998); defensiveness (Nyklicek, Vingerhoets, Van Heck, & Van Limpt, 1998); escapism (King et al., 1998); prayer (Ai, Peterson, & Boiling, 1997); pessimism (Powers & Jalowiec, 1987), and professional support (Erickson & Swain, 1990).

Cognitive and Physical

Coping strategies that fell under these domains included exercise (Ai et al., 1997; Ornish, Brown, Scherwitz, et al., 1990; Strain, 1996; Woodward, Berry, Rejeski, Ribisi, & Miller, 1994); diet (Ai et al.; Ornish et al.; Powers & Jalowiec, 1987; Strain); self-management (Lorig, 1996); stopping smoking (Ornish et al.); stress management (Ornish et al.; Powers & Jalowiec); medical treatment (Powers, & Jalowiec; Strain); seeking sympathy (Krogh et al., 1992); complementary therapy (Ai et al.), including folk remedies (Ai et al.; Strain).

Cognitive, Affective, and Physical

Empowerment is the strategy that uses all three areas of human functioning et al., 1997). Though the list of coping strategies used by individuals with health conditions associated with cardiovascular disease have been identified here, not all are deemed to be effective. Indeed, the following are said to be negative coping strategies that should be avoided: confrontive and avoidance behavior; defensiveness; escapism; pessimism; some types of social support; searching for a meaning, and taking or seeking out folk remedies (Feifel, Strack, & Nagy, 1987a; King et al., 1998; Nyklicek et al., 1998; Powers & Jalowiec, 1987; Strain, 1996).

Individual Factors Affecting Coping with Cardiovascular Disease

Hahn, Brooks, and Hartsough (1993) discovered that men with no blood pressure reactivity engaged in more emotion-focused coping strategies than men with blood pressure reactivity. This finding differs from the dominant view that emotion-focused coping is an ineffective coping strategy. It is thought that emotion-focused strategies such as venting may act as a catharsis for hypertensive patients, preventing a rise in blood pressure. Other individual factors included a greater use of escape-avoidance by subjects with high depressive symptoms (Landerville & Vezina, 1994).

Social Support for Coping with Cardiovascular Disease

In the main, social support was considered to be effective in coping with cardiovascular disease, predicting fewer depressive symptoms (Holahan, Moos, Holahan, & Brennan, 1995), faster remission times with higher levels of support (Koenig, 1998), and a reduced mortality with more social network ties. Patients with low levels of emotional support had twice the risk of death compared to those with more sources of support (Berckman & Austin, 1993).

Synthesis of Review: Coping Strategies for 11 Other Illnesses

The model just illustrated with cardiovascular disease was applied to each of the other 11 chronic diseases selected for our review. We have synthesized our findings to represent collectively the most frequently occurring coping strategies used with the 11 other chronic diseases of the 12 we selected. Through the collation of this evidence, we were able to identify some significant coping strategies that were common across all the disease states, although there was no substantial evidence for a particular priority among the most effective coping strategies in a given situation. We perceived this to be due to the individualistic nature of a patient's behavior and characteristics in adverse situations. Individuals cope in different ways, which may be from a naturalistic (genetic) framework, based on cultural norms and expectations, or from frequency of experience. What we were able to determine were the most frequently used strategies and those that were used at the onset of an illness such as stroke, diabetes mellitus, cancer, or vision or hearing impairment. Stroke, for instance, can occur with such speed and suddenness, affecting the patient in such a dramatic, disabling way, that it requires the immediate use of certain coping mechanisms. Other illnesses such as chronic obstructive pulmonary disease have a more insidious effect on the patient so that the coping strategies used are more adaptive to the progression of the disease.

Other Findings on Coping in the Literature

The following coping behaviors associated with the 11 diseases we selected are those identified most frequently in the literature in one or more domains.

Cognitive

Pain management that includes diversional therapy, visualization, and reinterpreting pain sensations (Gard, Harris, Edwards, & McCormack, 1988; Lin, 1998; Wilkie & Keefe, 1991); problem-solving (Endler, Courbasson, & Fillion, 1998; Landerville, Dube, Lalande, & Alain, 1994); information seeking (Clark et al., 1996; Norburn, Bernard, Konrad, & Woomert, 1995; Raleigh, 1992); adopting an optimistic behavior (Kalfoss, 1993); confrontive behavior (Feifel et al., 1987a; Kalfoss; Landerville et al., 1994; Michael, 1996); changing the situation (Kalfoss); maintaining control (De Ridder, Depla, Severens, & Malsch, 1997); mastery (Lorig et al., 1999); acceptance (Agrawal & Pandey, 1998; Koenig, 1988); drawing on past experiences (Kalfoss); supportant; making comparisons with others (Baker & Stern, 1993); self-reliant behavior (Landerville et al., 1994; Do Rozario, 1997) or self-blame (Bombardier, D'Amico, & Jordan, 1990; Kalfoss), and maintaining normality (Kalfoss; Robinson, 1993; Walker, Nail, Larsen, Magill, & Schwartz, 1996).

Affective

Demonstrating emotional response is key under this category, such as crying, daydreaming, denial, or anger (De Ridder et al., 1997; Eakes, 1993; Felton & Revenson, 1987; Kalfoss, 1993; Michael, 1996).

Physical

The use of assistive devices or technical aids (Fitzgerald & Parkes, 1998; Hallberg & Carisson, 1991; Scott, Lindberg, Melin, & Lyttkens, 1994).

Cognitive and Affective

Emotional (Bombardier et al., 1990; Clark et al., 1996; De Ridder et al., 1997; Koenig, Cohen, Blazer,& Pieper, 1992; Lehr & Kruse, 1992; Raleigh, 1992; Roberson, 1992); social and family support (Agrawal & Pandey, 1998; Bombardier et al.; Carruth & Boss, 1990; Clark et al., 1996; De Ridder et al.; Do Rozario, 1997; Koenig, 1998; Laferriere & Hamel Bissell, 1994; Landerville et al., 1994; Lehr & Kruse; Roberts et al., 1995; Rybarczyk, DeMarco, DelaCruz, & Lapidos, 1999); praying or having spiritual beliefs and having a sense of humor and a clear purpose in life (Halstead & Femsler, 1994). Other aspects cover evasive and fatalistic attitudes (De Ridder et al.), resignation (Degazon, 1995), and wish-fulfilling fantasy (Felton & Revenson, 1987)

Cognitive and Physical

Within these two categories are all aspects that embrace exercise regimens (Butler, Davis, Lewis, Nelson, & Strauss, 1998; Hickey, Wolf, Robins, Wagner, & Hank, 1995; Koenig, 1998; Morey et al., 1989; Shin,

1999; Stewart et al., 1994); yoga and relaxation methods (Hasitavej, 1995; Heidrich & Ryff, 1992; Hopman-Rock, Kraaimaat, Odding, & Bijisma, 1998; Lavery & Clarke, 1996; Lorig et al., 1999; Spiegel, 1999); assistive devices (Norburn et al., 1995); nutrition and diet control (Heidrich & Ryff); glucose monitoring (diabetes only) (Glasgow, Ruggiero, Eakin, Dryfoos, & Chobanian, 1997); compliance with medication (Shaul, 1995; Strain, 1996); palliative and folk remedies (Halstead & Femsler, 1994; Montbriand & Laing, 1991; Roberson, 1992); making behavioral changes, such as stopping smoking or cutting out alcohol (Koenig; Norburn et al.) and undertaking educational programs (Lacasse, Goldstein, & Guyatt, 1997; Petrie, 1990).

Cognitive, Affective, and Physical

Falling under these domains are empowerment (Arnold, Butler, Anderson, Funnell, & Feste, 1995; McDermott, 1995); psychosocial support (Clark et al., 1996; Heidrich & Ryff, 1992; Kalfoss, 1993; Koenig, 1998); stress reduction techniques and cognitive restructuring (Blake, Vandiver, Braun, Bertuso, & Straub, 1990); and aspects of palliative care interventions (Blake et al., DowneWamboldt & Melanson, 1995; Mahat, 1997).

Among this listing of coping strategies are some that had positive value and others that had a negative value when they were used to alleviate the effects of chronic illness. Those having positive results related to the patient who had high self-esteem and mastery of the situation (Penninx et al., 1998), who could engage in self-management activities (Baker & Stern, 1993), or who had inherent beliefs relating to cure or religious intents (Koenig et al., 1992; Scharloo et al., 1998). Those that were deemed more negative, or not recommended for use, included: confrontive behavior (Feifel et al., 1987a; Roberto, 1992); searching for meaning, avoidance, escapism (King et al., 1998); defensiveness (Nyklicek et al., 1998); pessimism, and certain types of social support (Powers & Jalowiec, 1987); fatalism (Herbert & Gregor, 1997; DownWamboldt & Melanson, 1995; Lavery & Clarke, 1996); taking abusive substances (Degazon, 1995); being emotive (DownWamboldt & Melanson; Halstead & Femsler, 1994); self-blame, (Parker et al., 1988; Revenson & Felton, 1989); withdrawal (Hopman-Rock et al., 1998); reinterpreting pain sensations and catastrophizing (Barkwell, 1991).

From the list of coping strategies that proved to be negative when used with chronic illnesses, there is evidence that certain ones are effective in some instances but not in others. For example, seeking social support can be either positive or negative, depending on the type of support and the circumstances for which it is used. For the most part, social support was identified within each disease entity as having a positive correlation and was written about copiously by a broad spectrum of scientific authors. This view was expressed more profoundly as the disease progressed towards a terminal point or when there were periods of acute exacerbation. Considering the perceived importance of social support as a coping strategy, it merits further discussion to best understand this phenomenon.

Social Support as a Means of Coping

Social support is well recognized in the literature as an effective means of coping in regard to stress and health needs. Often they are independently researched, however, which in the view of Schreurs and de Ridder (1997) fails to illustrate the relationship between them. In concurrence, Sarason, Sarason, and Pierce (1990) assert that the lack of a comprehensive theoretical framework prevents us from obtaining a clear view of the effect that social support has on health. Additionally, Coyne and DeLongis (1986) suggest that this lack of a theoretical framework hinders the argument that social support is always a supportive coping strategy. Coyne and DeLongis advanced the theory that social support has two main influences: the "buffering hypothesis" and the "main effect hypothesis." According to their buffering hypothesis, social support only has significant benefits for individuals who are experiencing the effects of a stressful event (Sherbourne, Meredith, Rogers, & Ware, 1992). Opponents of this stress-buffering model of support contend that it affects positive health outcomes associated with the activities of daily living, economic deprivation, psychosomatic symptoms, and emotional distress with older people (Arling, 1987; Revenson, Woliman, & Felton, 1983). On the other hand, the main-effect hypothesis is less challenging, in that it is conceptualized as social integration, which embraces feelings of stability, self-worth, and predictability. This view also recognizes the negative effects that social isolation and exclusion may have on health. Nonetheless, this should not always be an indicator of the efficacy of the coping mechanism but one that reflects the functional outcome of social integration.

Despite these opposing views on the efficacy of social support as a coping strategy, there is a plethora of evidence suggesting that there is a positive relationship between social support and health (Lopez & Mermeistein, 1987; Penninx et al., 1997; Ruberman, Weinblatt, Goldberg, & Chandhary, 1984; Seeman, Berkman, Kohout, et al., 1993). Welin, Larsson, Svardsudd, Tibbins, and Tiblin (1992) provide evidence also of the significance of social support in reducing the mortality and morbidity effects on individuals who have cancer, coronary heart disease, and coronary vascular disease. The mediating effect of social support with premature death is noteworthy, but other studies have shown that a lack of social support has a direct relationship with psychological distress and illness (Kaplan & Feinstain, 1974; Schaefer, Coyne, & Lazarus, 1981). However, this overriding attention to the positive nature of social support has been challenged. Stephens, Kinney, Norris, and Ritchie (1987) argue that it is necessary to identify the difference between positive and negative social interactions, and Coyne and Bolger (1990) believe that focusing on just the positive elements of social support distorts the truth and offers a romantic, idealized version.

The provision of social support is often grounded in a sense of duty by members of the nuclear family (Rook & Dooley, 1985) and incorporates the constructs of social expectations and social policy (Department of Health, 1989). The connotations of a "sense of duty" and "moral obligation" do not necessarily imply that support is always given willingly. Indeed, many kinds of long-sustained support during in a chronic health condition can cause feelings of resentment in the provider (Sarason et al., 1990). Furthermore, providing social support may serve as a source of additional income for some providers; conversely, some may incur costs that may be seen as a burden. Also, the premise that all providers of support have the requisite knowledge and skill to undertake the task competently may sometimes be inaccurate, in which case they could do more harm than good (Shumaker & Brownell, 1984). Some providers of social support have no understanding of their limitations and would boldly intervene regardless of the consequences of their actions. The balance of the relationship between provider and recipient can be combative in these sets of circumstances, and the independence (and choice) of the recipient may be ignored by the provider who asserts a dominant ("I know best") position. However, emotional, instrumental, or informational support from family and support from trusted friends is virtually always deemed to have a positive relationship.

Clearly, social support is a dynamic process that has to account for the differences in interpersonal relationships and different characteristics between the caregiver and the recipient, each of whom can be influenced by external variables. Similarly, Antonucci (1985) claims that social ties and relationships are never free of conflict, and suggests that support and conflict are juxtaposed and are a feature of everyday reality in caregiving. To gain a clearer understanding of the various nuances of social support requires further research, particularly in relation to the benefits for the older person who is coping with multiple health conditions.

Effects of the Most Frequently Occurring Comorbidities

By exploring the literature from a single-disease perspective in a structured manner, it was easy to establish some important effects of the most frequently encountered comorbidities. Indeed the relationship between cardiovascular disease and diabetes mellitus was found to be well documented, highlighting key areas of the interrelatedness of the two disease states. Chief among these was the fact that the progression and management of these diseases are instrumental in order to promote health maintenance, aid restoration of health when an acute exacerbation of one of the diseases occurred, support and prevent emotional distress and clinical depression that would impair cognitive ability, and prevent social exclusion and social isolation. If either of these two disease entities is managed in isolation from the other, then the efficacy of coping is marginalized and can have disastrous results in speeding the disease towards a terminal outcome and in increasing the dependency of the patient on caregivers and the state.

The interrelationship of cardiovascular disease and diabetes mellitus to health conditions arising out of mismanagement or lack of recognition of another disease entity is similarly depicted with other comorbid relationships. For instance, it is evident that cardiovascular disease on its own presents the patient with health problems that require adaptive coping strategies or behavioral changes or both. Nonetheless, the situation is compounded when the patient has another disease such as chronic obstructive pulmonary disease. COPD presents the older adult with a set of health conditions that lead to hypoxia (oxygen deprivation) or hypercapnia (carbon dioxide retention), or both, which increases with the progress of the disease and results in a decreased cognitive functioning capacity. This situation in turn affects the patient's problem-solving ability, motor coordination, or memorization function (Frazer, Leicht, & Baker, 1996). Memory failure will inevitably reduce the older person's ability to comply with the medication regimen that is essential to maintain cardiovascular output. Given these sets of circumstances, the older patient's anxiety levels increase, which can further traumatize the capacity of their heart to function effectively and further reduce the lung function with regard to oxygen exchange. This cyclical process of events, if unchanged, leads to a rapid deterioration of health and a reduced capacity to maintain independence of living and quality of life (Felton & Revenson, 1987. Though this phenomenon is related to cardiovascular disease and COPD, the picture is just as grim when there is a combination of cardiovascular disease and stroke. Stroke invariably leaves the patient with some degree of physical and cognitive impairment, restricting their capacity to undertake activities of daily living independently (Hodgson, 1998). Such incidents affect the treatment of the concomitant cardiovascular disease because activity levels rapidly decline.

Symptoms of pain, such as those associated with arthritis, can be particularly debilitating; indeed, arthritis is one of the major diseases of the older population and reduces their mobility. Consequently, if a patient has not only a progressive arthritic condition but also suffers from cardiovascular disease, the ability to cope effectively is greatly impaired. Acute pain counteracts any mental capacity to cope with a host of health conditions arising from the two diseases. Conversely, if the cardiovascular disease is at an advanced stage, there is greater probability that mobility will be further reduced. This situation limits the person with arthritis, who is encouraged to move to his or her optimum capacity in order to prevent further stiffness of the joints and to manage the effects of acute and chronic pain.

When an older person suffers from a stroke, there is evidence that the risk of falls resulting in fractures also greatly increases. Reduced mobility is an obvious risk factor (Hodgson, 1998), but it can also be associated with previously undetected osteoporosis. Bed rest enforced by a fracture leads to muscular atrophy, cardiovascular deconditioning, and loss of flexibility. The short- and long-term effects of such competing health problems can, and most often do, lead to disability, depression, social isolation, and helplessness.

Although visual and hearing impairments in the older adult are not life threatening, they are worthy of note because they can have a significant impact on the ability of the patient to effectively cope with other health conditions. Individuals who have visual impairment are at risk for frequent falls and resultant fractures (Dargent Molina, Hays, & Breart, 1996). Conversely, impaired hearing and visual ability may render an older person more susceptible to accidents. Bone fractures create the need for bed rest, which further adds to health problems if another disease such as diabetes is present, which can result in a decreased glucose tolerance (Rader & Vaughen, 1994), reduced cardiorespiratory and muscular functioning, and flexibility. Health is further compromised with vision impairment due to the inability to recognize medications or to read labels that are needed to help manage other comorbid diseases.

Depression and the Coping Relationship

Depression has an identified comorbid relationship with other chronic disease states in the older person (Evans, Copeland, & Dewey, 1991; Katona et al., 1999) and prevents effective coping strategies from being deployed (Evans et al.; Landerville & Vezina, 1994). Research also indicates that some chronic health conditions are more strongly related to depressive symptoms than to others (Penninx et al., 1996). Having two or more chronic health conditions is known to increase the risk of depression (Angel & Angel, 1995; Bazargan, 1996; Burnette & Mui, 1994; Lyness, Duberstein, King, Cox, & Cain, 1999; Palinkas, Wingard, & Barrett Connor, 1990; Roberts, Kaplan, Shema, & Strawbridge, 1997; Vandelisdonk, Furer, Kroonen, & Marijnissen, 1992). The level of depression varies and increases in the older person if there is impairment in independent activities of daily living (Alexopoulos et al., 1996) or disability from increased physical dysfunction, which result in the loss of independence. If depressive symptoms are assessed and treated within the context of the chronic disease, then it is reported that patients who are more active in their coping behaviors have a better effect (Rosenberg, Peterson, & Hayes, 1987).

Coping with Pain

Pain is a complex subjective experience, incorporating sensory, emotional, and cognitive components, which makes its measurement very difficult. The control of pain is an issue for many chronically ill patients but is of particular concern to patients who have arthritis or cancer, and many patients regard pain as an index of disease severity. Other psychological factors such as anxiety, suggestion, attention, and conditioning render the psychological treatment of chronic pain less effective (Fry & Wong, 1991). Treatment with psychological interventions is recommended to prevent the development of a passive and helpless role, often associated with medical therapies in which dependence is encouraged.

Strategies for coping with pain and managing pain can be undertaken, including trying to function in spite of the pain, distracting oneself from the pain or its progression, and through muscular relaxation. These cognitive coping strategies require continuous effort by the patient in order for them to be effective. They also require patients to have confidence in their ability to manage the pain through their own coping strategies and personal resources. Older people tend to use fewer cognitive coping strategies, but often use external coping strategies such as medication (Herbert & Gregor, 1997), transcutaneous electrical nerve stimulation units, or heat treatment (Lin, 1998; Strain, 1996).

The ability of chronically ill persons to withstand pain and reduce its impact on their lifestyle depends on their psychological coping abilities. Fry and Wong (1991) found that problem-focused interventions were more beneficial than emotion-focused interventions for reducing pain ratings in a cohort of older subjects with chronic knee pain. The superiority of problem-focused coping in the management of pain is thought to be the result of an increase in perceived control and competence. Passive, emotion-focused coping includes the tendency to depend on others for pain control, to engage in wishful thinking, and to restrict functioning because of pain.

Other pain coping strategies include those that are seen to be adaptive, assimilative, and accommodative. Adaptive pain coping strategies include behavioral efforts to ease the pain as well as cognitive processes such as distracting oneself from the pain, reinterpreting or ignoring the pain sensations, and making positive self statements about one's ability to manage pain. Assimilation methods are characterized by active attempts to maintain goals by altering the situation. Accommodative coping strategies involve neutralizing goal discrepancies by downgrading personal standards, reorienting toward new feasible goals, and generally being more flexible by adjusting desires or preferences. Fry and Wong (1991) contend that patients are more likely to learn coping strategies that are consistent with their preferred style, implying that interventions are likely to be ineffective if they do not comply with individual choice of coping strategy. Attention to a preferred coping style is therefore an important consideration by health care professionals in their health assessment and case management of older people with multiple chronic health conditions.

Toward a Theory on the Effects of Coping on Comorbidity

Throughout our exploration and synthesis of the literature relating to comorbidity and coping, it is clear that there has been little discourse to provide a theory on the effects of coping styles and strategies on multiple chronic health conditions. In the absence of such a theory, we have designed a template for such discourse, based on direct evidence from the literature. Our model considers these questions:

1. What is known about coping with chronic disease in general?
2. What is known about individual-specific, disease-specific, and social-specific variables in coping with stressors in old age?
3. What is known about the more frequent combinations of diseases and their impact on patients?
4. What is known about the effect of comorbidity on other patient-related outcomes such as quality of life, activities of daily living, and disability (Fried et al., 1999)?

Based on these related and interrelated concepts of known entities, it is apparent that there are different parameters within which coping may be affected by comorbidity. Schellevis, van der Velden, van de Lisdonk, van Eijk, and van Weel (1993) provide a conceptual framework for comorbidity in the specific domain of coping strategies for comorbidities, whose conceptualizations we have revised as follows:

• *Concurrence.* The use of individual coping strategies associated with one particular condition alongside unrelated coping strategies associated with one or more comorbid conditions
• *Clustering.* The increased prevalence of certain combinations of conditions beyond what might be expected by chance but which cannot be easily attributed to the contributing conditions themselves
• *Causality.* Where coping strategies have been established as prominent for two or more individual diseases and are significantly present in comorbid states of these diseases when in combination
• *Disease-Specific.* Where the characteristic coping strategies associated with a particular disease are also associated with that disease when found in combination with other conditions, to the extent that they subsume or obscure the coping strategies that might be expected to occur in these comorbid conditions

These concepts may nicely outline a simplistic framework with which to explain the various relationships of coping with comorbidity, but they fail to augment the complex behavioral reactions to disease. Such complex phenomena must be explained beyond a classification that assumes a direct cause-and-effect relationship between conditions and strategies. Therefore, there is a need to add to the model of Schellevis et al. such factors as the temporal nature of the diseases involved, their respective trajectories of illness, the recency of their onset, their severity, and their perceived importance to the patient (regardless of the clinical manifestation or health outcome). Working within these constructs, we designed a model for analysis of both written secondary data from the literature and for primary data collected for the purpose of our project. Our model reflects five dimensions that represent the different directions of the effects of the comorbidities.

1. *The Additive Effect.* This dimension would assume that adding comorbidity to disease A would result in corresponding strategies A1 + B1. Thus, a parallel can be drawn with research into the effect of comorbidity on disability where the question has been asked, Does disability rise linearly with the number of chronic conditions? (Young, 1994). Variations on this include (a) where the coping strategies are again added but where some form of prioritization or filtering takes place ($A1/x + B1/x$ where x represents a threshold beyond which the patient cannot entertain or tolerate further strategies); and (b) where the coping strategies for two diseases are similar enough to merely reinforce or strengthen the direction of effect (Ab + Ba).

2. *The Multiplicative Effect.* Conceptually this dimension is very similar to the additive effect just described. However, the difference here is one of degree. Instead of a direct correspondence between coping strategies for the two individual diseases and the coping strategy for the disease interaction, one would observe an effect that is even greater. This model is supported by the findings of the study by Fried et al. (1999), who point out that having two diseases was associated with a substantially higher risk of disability than is expected by combining the individual disease effects. Again the question has been asked in the context of comorbidity and its effect on the disability: Is the relationship exponential? (Young, 1994). The concept of synergism often applies in this context (Young; Fried et al.).

3. *The Modifying Effect.* This dimension would assume that adding comorbidity B to disease A does not merely lead to coping strategies

that are the sum of the coping strategies for the individual diseases. Instead, the interaction of the two diseases leads to one being dominant in terms of governing the coping strategies and the other merely adding subordinate strategies determined by the secondary condition. The implication is that the secondary condition would have an abbreviated or curtailed coping strategy because of a focus on the main disorder $(A1 + B1/x)$. The dominance of the main disease could be from the point of view of (a) longest duration or (b) perceived severity.

4. *The Counteractive Effect.* Both of the previous scenarios assume that the coping strategies for the two diseases are similar in their direction of effect, and so the influence of both is discernible, even when some of the individual effect is filtered or curtailed. In an opposing scenario, a coping strategy that is a natural choice for condition A is not apparent because of a counteractive effect from the coping strategy for condition B $(B1 - A1)$. This may be at a practical level where the coping strategy for a new condition (either through novelty or severity) completely obscures the previous coping strategy for the single disorder A, or it may be at a psychological level (where denial of the severity of the new condition B leads to a disproportionate focus on coping strategies for the more minor condition A) $(A1 - B1)$.

5. *The Interactive Effect.* This type of effect would be characterized by more successful coping. Either the patient is able to switch between coping strategies for conditions as and when required (A1:B1: A1:B1, etc.), or the patient comes to view the composite condition as a single entity requiring a tailored (individualistic) coping strategy in its own right $(C1 = A1*B1)$. This latter circumstance is again modeled by the Fried et al. (1999) study, where one of two diseases is associated with disability only in the presence of the other single disease. The disease interaction can therefore be properly classified as a single entity, for example, arthritis-stroke or arthritis-hearing.

Further expansion of this hypothetical model can be explored using the frameworks of definition, interaction, and observation, and through research findings of comorbidities that offer hypothetical examples as well as sample statements made by patients that might indicate a coping effect. Thus, extending the discourse with additional considerations within the framework of these five dimensions can more fully explain the complexities of the efficacy of coping with multiple health problems. For example, within the *Additive Effect,* three subtypes can be examined: aggregative, assimilative, and reinforcing. Each subtype considers the aspect of coping with comorbidity, but from different parameters and perspectives. There are two subtypes for the *Modifying Effect,* adaptive and primacy, and two subtypes for the *Counteractive Effect,* transferal and denial. The *Interactive Effect* embraces the subtypes of crossover and sublimation. The following illustrate the hypothetical research findings and likely patient statements for each subtype:

• *Aggregative.* The patient may have coronary heart disease with arthritis, which independently contributes to disability, but this particular comorbidity also places individuals at increased risk when a new disease event occurs. Thus, there may be an interaction between prevalent disease and incident, or new onset disease in causing disability.

The patient with arthritis and visual impairment would say, "I cope by taking NSAIDS for my arthritis and using the banister to make sure that I don't trip while walking down the poorly lit stairs."

• *Assimilative.* There is an underlying assumption that all cumulative diseases are perceived as equally important to the patient. The hypothetical research study would establish general congruence between the coping strategies for individual diseases and for the comorbid conditions when observed together. However, an incomplete picture would pertain with subsidiary coping strategies not being in the comorbid state.

The patient using such an approach to coping would probably say, "I just concentrate on my exercises for my heart disease and my insulin injections for my diabetes, but apart from that I just continue as normal."

• *Reinforcement.* This characteristic is seen when the coping strategies for two diseases are similar enough to merely reinforce or strengthen the direction of effect. In this sense it could be hypothesized that this might be the case with the comorbid occurrence of osteoporosis and arthritis that, according to Roberto (1989), occurs in 71.3% of osteoporosis sufferers.

The patient would probably say, "Since I have had osteoporosis as well as arthritis, I find that I won't move at all unless there is someone around to help me."

• *Adaptive.* The dominance of the "indexed disease" would in this subtype relate to the condition of longest duration. Here the coping strategy is based on the longest standing condition with only minor concessions to new conditions. The hypothetical research findings would be seen where the primary findings of a coping scale match those for a single disease, but where the patient adds specific strategies to assist in coping with a secondary condition.

The patient statement representing a long-standing chronic obstructive pulmonary disease and recent onset arthritis might be, "When I have a sudden attack of breathlessness, I have to go and get my oxygen, but since my arthritis I have had the cylinder mounted on wheels so that I am able to maneuver it more easily."

• *Primacy.* The indexed disease is determined by its perceived severity. The importance of the expression "perceived" is illustrated by a study examining lay explanations of illness (Strain, 1996). An example of the primacy subset emphasizes how a new condition can modify previous coping behavior in that a patient who is struggling to function with severe pulmonary or coronary heart disease may compensate to the point of incapacitation with something as relatively benign as an ankle sprain (Berman & Studenski, 1998).

The patient would say something like this: "Well, of course I managed to lead a normal life despite my arthritis. However, when I sprained my ankle I couldn't be expected to get things done, so I just resigned myself to being waited on hand and foot."

• *Transfer.* This subset operates at a practical level, where the coping strategy for a new condition (either through novelty or severity) completely obscures the previous coping strategy for the single disorder. The hypothetical research findings would identify a coping scale that would only pick up the characteristics of a primary disorder, although further qualitative feedback may reveal additional complicating co-morbidities.

The patient might say, "Now that I am partially sighted, I tend to get much closer to people I meet or to the television, and I find that this helps me to be able to hear them better so I can overcome my hearing difficulties."

• *Denial model.* This model operates at the psychological level, where denial of the severity of the new condition B leads to a disproportionate focus on coping strategies for the more minor condition A. Under these circumstances the patient would deny the more severe condition. The hypothetical research findings, using a coping scale with a patient with a stroke, might find that they focus exclusively on unrelated hearing or vision difficulties and pay no attention to their mobility or language difficulties.

The patient would probably say, "No I don't have any problems with my heart—after all, that heart attack was nearly a decade ago. But what gets me down is now my eyesight is going. I miss the chance to play tennis with my grandchildren and we have to play soccer instead."

• *Crossover.* The interactive type of effect would be characterized by more successful coping. The patient would be able to switch between coping strategies for conditions as and when required. Such an approach to coping strategies would be very difficult to establish from a single administration of a coping measurement tool. The hypothetical research findings would illustrate that a coping scale administered to patients several weeks apart would find completely different profiles, first resembling one disease, then another.

The patient would likely say, "Well if you had only been here last week you would have found me complaining about my arthritis, but this week it is much better, so I've just got my breathing to worry about."

• *Sublimation.* Under these conditions a coping strategy would be almost unrecognizable from among individual coping strategies for each contributing condition. It would appear rather as a new coping model specifically adapted for the purpose of coping with the comorbidity. The hypothetical research finding would have a coping scale in which the results bear little relation to those of someone with one or another of the contributing conditions. It would probably detect a coping strategy that has become strongly predominant.

The patient would say, "Well once it became clear that my heart attack and my asthma had put an end to my jogging, I threw myself body and soul into the local bridge club, which I am now chairing, and I am playing for my city next week."

It is hoped that these hypotheses will be explored and tested in future research. However, other factors that pertain to coping with chronic multiple health conditions need further exploration. For instance, there are coping strategies that operate at a symptom level (e.g., coping with breathlessness), or at a systemic level (e.g., a coping strategy targeted at a number of manifestations of the same underlying disease process, such as diabetes and associated complications of neuropathy, retinopathy, etc.), or at the more epidemiological level where there is "pure" coexistence of identifiable disease entities, that is, where two diseases occur in the same patient.

Conclusions

Our review has been exhaustive, showing that there is a paucity of literature on older adults coping with multiple chronic health conditions that meets all of our criteria. Although many authors have demonstrated an interest in all types of coping strategies across the whole spectrum of chronic diseases, they have not been concerned with multiple health conditions. Fried et al. (1999) provide useful data on the occurrence of comorbidities and their effects on disability but made no attempt to relate this information to requirements for coping. After exploring 7,900 references taken from 12 different sources, the review team did not find one article where coping with comorbidity in older adults was a major focus. Therefore, to tease out the evidence of effective coping models, we changed direction to explore the literature that had focused on coping with a *single* chronic disease in our attempt to compile a framework of understanding. The process of our investigation involved

1. A detailed investigation of the cognitive, affective, and physical effects of 12 key diseases, from which we were able to identify the impact of principal comorbidities;
2. A detailed investigation of coping instruments and coping strategies as demonstrated with reference to these 12 key diseases;
3. An examination of the theoretical literature in connection with comorbidity, including psychological models, in an attempt to identify appropriate theoretical constructs of direct applicability to the context of coping;
4. A construction of a new theoretical model of comorbidity with specific reference to coping strategies.

On completion of the review, we were able to identify coping strategies used within a single disease classification, those that were most frequently used, and those that were not used often. The efficacy of these coping behaviors was identified as either positive or negative, and by analyzing and synthesizing this information we were able to hypothesize the effect of comorbidity on coping and make the following recommendations for clinical practice, education, and future research.

Recommendations for Clinical Practice

It is evident that coping with any chronic health condition is a considerable challenge, but when it is compounded by several competing chronic health conditions, then the situation is very different and requires a degree of problem solving and greater understanding from the individual and the professional body as a whole. For example, reducing health conditions into discrete and isolated functions is not a model that explains or supports the multiplicity and complex phenomena associated with coping with comorbidity. This requires a different perspective that draws on the paradigms of holism, recognizing that people *are* the sum of their parts. On the contrary, holism considers that the health of each person is maintained by their individual makeup and the interconnectedness of their bodily functions, emotions, belief systems, social connections and support systems, and the environment. Therefore, coping models must address this issue if efficacy of coping with multiple chronic health conditions is to be achieved. Of central importance to meeting this challenge is sensitivity to the individual's perspective. Addressing this concept is the key principle for promoting effective coping strategies that when deployed can ameliorate the effects of multiple chronic health conditions. In considering this point, health care professionals must assess individuals from their unique characteristics and from a holistic perspective. A plan of action should empower the person, and their significant caregivers, to use effective coping strategies that can be adapted and personalized to accommodate the individual's changed and constantly changing needs throughout the life span of the chronic disease process.

Applying Effective Interventions

To be able to assist and advise the older person to effectively cope with comorbidity, health care professionals must have a comprehensive understanding of interventions that promote effective coping. On examination of the literature, broad ranges of interventions have been documented with a prominent focus on the following areas:

Education

Education offers support and encourages self-management and participation in self-help groups. These approaches encourage learning that assists older adults with maintaining independence, but at the same time provide effective and meaningful social support. In addition, health promoting activities seem to have the contributing effect of empowering the individual to increase their knowledge and understanding with respect to the need to comply with treatment in order to prevent short-term and long-term complications. The most prominent health-promoting activities cited are diet, exercise, medication, and informational support.

Social Support

Social support and social networks were found to be significant factors in the efficacy of coping with multiple health conditions over a sustained period of time. Notwithstanding this fact, the literature suggests that as people age, they are more likely to have progressive multiple chronic health conditions, and their social support and networks diminish accordingly. It is therefore imperative for health care professionals to address this issue by encouraging involvement with organized activities and formalizing support structures for the individual from voluntary or statutory services. Of particular note is the apparent need for the older person to address their spirituality, which is often extolled in the literature as having a positive relationship with a person's better physical and mental health and well-being. This benefit is possibly related to an increased social network when attending religious services, or having a shared experience with others who have a similar belief system.

Empowerment

Empowering individuals was mentioned in the previous section on education, but it is of significant importance on its own. The term *empowerment* itself implies a common understanding, but when the literature is examined, it is just as complex and misunderstood as is the concept of comorbidity (Basford, Nyatanga, & Dann, 2001). Regardless of this observation, it is necessary for health care professionals to recognize the various empowerment models that can be employed in order to help an individual gain or regain control over their chronic condition, and, thereby maintain some degree of independence.

Chief among these empowerment strategies are those that engage the person to use active, problem-focused methods rather than passive emotion-focused ones. Emotion-focused coping strategies on the other hand, may, allow an outward expression of anger that can be seen as positive, rather than suppressed anger that may manifest in further physiological dysfunction (e.g., hypertension), or conversely, when the situation presents little opportunity for beneficial change or is of brief duration. Other personal characteristics, such as flexibility, are viewed positively, particularly when the chronic condition is associated with frequent flare-ups and downturns.

To date, much reference has been made to the importance of social support and social networks. But there is a negative side to social support, particularly if the individual is made to feel disempowered by the provider. Given this fact, individuals need to be taught how to identify negative sources of social support and engage in those that promote effective coping strategies.

Encouraging individuals to become more empowered is seen as a positive outcome for effectively coping with multiple chronic health conditions. However, empowering individuals also means recognizing the unique characteristics that lead them to become more empowered. For example, persons with a strong internal locus of control, those who have a hardy nature and relate more comfortably to problem-solving approaches, and those who generally have an optimistic outlook on life are the best candidates for using empowerment strategies.

Therapeutic Interventions

Multiple chronic health conditions often require the older person to take medical prescriptions to maintain or restore their health. Most often, there is no cure for their multiple health conditions, and management requires taking prescribed drugs in the manner and times indicated by their health care provider over a long and sustained period. Successful management requires the individual to adhere to the regimen if complications are to be avoided, not an easy task for an older person, particularly if there is no perceived benefit. Further, there is sometimes no recognition of the contraindications of certain prescribed drugs that can have an adverse effect on a person's well-being and overall health improvement. Many older persons with chronic illnesses are increasingly turning to complementary modalities without consulting with their regular health care professionals. Although using alternative remedies may not in themselves be dangerous, they can cause adverse reactions when taken simultaneously with prescribed medication. It is a phenomenon that health care professionals must have knowledge about and be able to advise clients about, based on the best possible evidence.

Educating Health Care Professionals

The education of health care professionals should not be undertaken in isolation from one another, given the need for the older person with multiple chronic health conditions to seek help and guidance from a range of professional groups over a sustained period of time. Failures in health care provision often occur due to the lack of coordinated, well communicated approaches to care, or to the lack of professional understanding of therapeutic interventions used by different health care disciplines.

A good command of the definitions of coping strategies and a comprehensive understanding of the term *comorbidity* are pivotal to any health professional's education on coping with multiple chronic health conditions by the older person. Health professionals need to have a knowledge and understanding of coping strategies used with symptoms rather than with specific diseases and of the various therapeutic interventions (orthodox and complementary) that require a range of different coping strategies that may not always be sympathetic to one another. Last but not least, health professionals need to recognize individual differences and to be more discerning with regard to the interrelationship of physical, psychological, spiritual, social, and environmental influences that foster effective coping with chronic illness.

Recommendations for Further Research

At face value there appeared to be a plethora of research in the field of coping with multiple chronic health conditions by older persons, yet this systematic review has revealed quite the opposite. The most important bias identified in the quantitative literature is the preponderance of attention to the disease rather than to the individual. Although the qualitative literature does explore the phenomenon of the individual within social constructs, more study is needed. Instead of focusing on large numbers of individuals with a specific disease and how they have coped with that disease, individual and social parameters need to be examined in relation to coping with disease symptoms. A major benefit of this report is the inclusion of both qualitative and quantitative data, which we have attempted to combine in order to reach a comprehensive understanding of how older adults cope with multiple chronic illnesses. This led to the development of a comorbidity and social support model, which is meant to foster understanding of the development of effective coping strategies used with comorbidity.

Much of the literature has concerned itself with single-disease self-management models. However, it is clear that their applicability to those with multiple health conditions can be argued through extrap-olation of findings rather than by direct evidence. In addition, the question remains of whether these models can be usefully translated to other disease settings than the one for which they were developed. Compounding this challenge is the fact that the literature on coping is largely psychological, while the comorbidity literature has emerged from an epidemiological bias. Interdisciplinary models need to be developed that use both quantitative and qualitative frameworks to examine coping strategies used with comorbidity from a holistic perspective.

In essence, further research is also required to explore lay explana-tions and understanding of comorbid conditions as a means of ad-dressing self-management from an individualistic position. Then a consistent model can be derived, using individual explanations drawn from personal experience. For instance, it is necessary to examine the extent to which individuals explain different health problems in the same way and in conjunction with each other.

Refining and Validating Instruments

Within the field of research on coping with comorbidity, tools and instruments have frequently been adapted and amended without due consideration of their validity and reliability. It is imperative that the scientific community develop new ways through which meaningful information can be explored that will better illustrate the efficacy of models that can aid coping with comorbidity. There is a need to ex-plore health problems from the symptomological perspective rather than from a disease-specific approach. Further, examinations of ther-apeutic interventions (orthodox and complementary) need to be ex-plored, as do the inclusion criteria for clinical trials that may exclude persons with comorbid conditions. It is paramount that researchers in this field acknowledge that comorbidity prevents a reductionistic, clean examination of the facts, but that it is nonetheless important to gain information by being creative and innovative with the development of new models and instruments.

The challenge for us as researchers is to validate our hypothetical frameworks through the perceptions of those living with multiple chronic health conditions, their formal caregivers, and those provid-ing informal support function—whereas the challenge for practitio-ners is to change clinical practice and gain knowledge and understanding through education.

Acknowledgments

This systematic review was the first phase of the research grant awarded by the AARP Andrus Research Foundation, which was followed by the second phase conducted at the Pennsylvania State University. The principal investigator was Leonard W. Poon, PhD. The co–principal investigator and project manager for phase one was Lynn Basford. The co–principal investigator and project manager for phase two was Sarah Hall Gueldner, PhD. Clare Dowzer was the research associate. The consultant and co–project manager for phase one was Andrew Booth, and the literature search assistant was Sue James.

Chapter 9

Managing Multiple Chronic Health Conditions in Everyday Life

Janice Penrod, Sarah Hall Gueldner, and Leonard W. Poon

Typically, health issues faced in middle and older adulthood are *chronic* in nature. Hoffman, Rice, and Sung (1996) estimated that 88% of older adults in the United States were affected by at least one chronic condition and that 69% lived with more than one chronic condition. These conditions are not curable; rather, they are lifelong concerns that often require changes in lifestyle patterns to manage or control symptoms and potentially life-threatening sequela. Beyond lifestyle, chronic conditions extend into multiple facets of life, including role function, perceptions of the self, and the ability to act independently (Miller, 1992).

Living with multiple conditions creates a complex interplay of symptoms, concerns, and management strategies collectively described as comorbidity. For the purposes of this discussion, comorbidity is any combination of diseases, conditions, malfunctions, or injury symptoms, as described by Kraemer (1995). Coping, defined by Newman (1990) as "any action/cognition which takes place in relation to the disease or illness" (p. 161), provides a holistic perspective of the collective conditions and strategies employed by older adults as they go through daily life while confronting their multiple chronic health conditions.

The exploratory study reported in this chapter was designed to further our understanding of the effects of comorbidity on the daily lives of active, socially engaged older adults. We believe that an *emic* perspective (that is, the view of those who are actually living with comorbidity) provides essential baseline knowledge about this complex phenomenon. Thus, this preliminary research investigated the ecology of coping with multiple chronic health conditions and provides fertile ground for further research into this complex life experience. Our goal in future research is to develop an efficient assessment guide that holistically integrates an understanding of coping strategies used by older adults facing multiple conditions; and subsequently, to suggest practical interventions that bolster the older adult's use of successful strategies and expand their repertoire of effective strategies in order to maximize health in the face of chronicity.

This chapter describes and discusses our initial investigation of the way older adults manage their chronic health conditions and the associated consequences of comorbidities in everyday life. First, a screening survey designed to ascertain the self-reported incidence and perceived impact of 11 chronic conditions is discussed. Next, the methods and findings of focus groups exploring the experiences and strategies used by these older adults to get through daily life with multiple chronic conditions are presented. In the third section, a process-oriented model, Staying in Control, conceptually describes the ecology of living with comorbidity experienced by this sample. Finally, the chapter concludes with a brief discussion of what we've learned from this sample and what we have yet to explore in order to understand better the personal experience of living with comorbidity.

Screening Survey: Establishing Comorbidity and Perceived Impact

Following approval by a university office of regulatory compliance for human subjects research, our initial study consisted of a screening survey that documented the self-report of chronic conditions and a rating of the impact of these conditions on day-to-day living. The survey was administered to a purposefully selected sample of socially engaged, community-dwelling older adults in order to explore examples of successful coping. The findings of the survey were then used to establish a sampling frame to theoretically segment the composition of focus groups according to number of conditions, impact rating, age, and gender.

Survey Development

The survey format was designed to establish the existence of comorbidity (defined as two or more reported chronic conditions) and to differentiate between participants' awareness of the conditions and their actually taking action to address these conditions. Brief demographics were collected, including age and gender, for the purpose of focus group segmentation and for acquiring the contact information needed to solicit participation in subsequent group discussions. The survey items related to reported chronic conditions were based on a question stem that read: Has your doctor ever told you that you have any of the following conditions?

Following this stem, the 11 chronic conditions were listed for the older adults to rate. Health conditions were cited using common language rather than medical terminology in order to enhance the older adults' comprehension of the items. The chronic conditions included in the screening survey, in the order in which they were presented is as follows:

- Heart trouble
- Arthritis
- High blood pressure
- Diabetes
- Hearing problems
- Lung problems
- Osteoporosis
- Problems with vision
- Urinary or bladder problems
- Cancer
- Stroke

Ten of the 11 conditions on this list were selected based on findings from the literature search reported by Poon, Basford, Dowzer, and Booth in chapter 7 of this book. The research team added urinary and bladder problems to assess the impact of incontinence, urgency, and frequency due to the known clinical impact of these conditions among older adult populations. Because this listing was not exhaustive, participants were given the opportunity to write in and rate up to three additional conditions.

Impact was conceptually defined as the degree to which the older adult thinks about or acts upon a condition in daily life, and was

Table 9.1 Impact Rating Scale

Assigned value	Response
0	No, my doctor never mentioned this to me.
1	Yes, but I don't think much about it.
2	Yes, I pay attention to my treatment, but I don't think about it too much.
3	Yes, I think about it pretty often and I pay close attention to my treatment.
4	Yes, I think about it nearly all the time and do all I can to feel better or get through the day.

captured using a 4-point scale. Table 9.1 shows the 4-point Impact Rating Scale developed for this purpose.

A panel of experts ($n = 10$) consisting of physicians and nurses who work closely with older adults reviewed the survey to confirm content validity. In addition, the survey was pilot tested by older adults ($n = 5$) for clarity of instructions, legibility of print and format, ease of administration, and approximate time for completion. No revisions were deemed necessary following these reviews.

Sample

Because this study focused on successful coping, the sample was purposefully directed toward active, engaged older adults. Subjects who were mobile, cognitively intact, and able to manage independent community living were recruited through a senior membership program at a community hospital in the northeastern United States. Inclusion criteria for initial participation in the screening survey were broadly defined as being aged 55 or older and participating in a health-related social-educational event. Attendance at such an event was used as a proxy for measurement of the subject's cognitive status; that is, participation in the social-educational event was deemed to indicate adequate cognitive functioning for possible inclusion in subsequent small group discussions. Then, based on the findings of the survey, additional inclusion criteria were developed for focus group segmentation (discussed later in this chapter).

Members of the research team attended the previously scheduled educational events to give a brief overview of the project and solicit participation. Signed informed consent—worded to include both the survey and, if applicable, participation in small group discussions—was explained and obtained. Instructions for completing the screening survey and a sample item were then read aloud. Those choosing to participate completed the survey on-site prior to attending the educational program.

Finding

The derived sample (n = 122) was 79.5% women and 20.5% men. The average age of participants was 70 years, with a range of 55 through 88 years. On average, this sample reported four chronic conditions (range 0–12 conditions) with a mean impact rating of 2.26 for all reported conditions. Frequency and mean impact ratings for each listed and written-in condition are displayed in Table 9.2.

Despite expectations of increasing numbers of chronic conditions with increasing age, no significant correlation (or curvilinear effect) was demonstrated between age and number of health conditions in this sample. Further, given the same number of health conditions, no significant differences of perceived impact were found among the three different age segments (young-old, aged 55–64; middle-old, aged 65–74; and old-old, aged 75–88), except among those with either heart problems or high blood pressure, although there was a tendency toward lower perceived impact of these problems as age increased ($p \leq .06$).

Factor analysis revealed that clusters of conditions frequently occurred, including heart trouble, hypertension, and stroke; arthritis, lung problems, and osteoporosis; hearing problems, urinary problems, and diabetes; and cancer and vision problems. The total number of reported health conditions was positively correlated with the average impact ascribed to each existing condition ($p < .05$) and the average impact across all conditions ($p < .001$).

Though bivariate analysis revealed no significant difference between men's and women's perceived impact of conditions, findings of multivariate analysis examining a model in which age *and* gender could be interacting to influence perceived impact produced significant findings. Age was a significant predictor of impact of chronic conditions for men ($p < .01$), but not for women. Overall, older men perceived the impact of their conditions to be greater than did younger men. This trend was not supported among women; in fact, perception of impact steadily decreased with age in women (although it was not statistically significant).

Table 9.2 Frequency of Reported Conditions and Mean Impact Rating per Condition

Condition	Frequency of report (%)	Mean impact rating
Arthritis	64	2.51
Vision problems	64	2.15
High blood pressure	52	2.42
Heart trouble	41	2.37
Urinary/bladder problems	36	2.38
Hearing problems	25	2.13
Osteoporosis	23	2.21
Cancer	23	1.96
Lung problems	22	2.13
Diabetes	19	2.68
Stroke	12	2.08
Additional conditions:		
Gastrointestinal concerns	12	3.14
Musculoskeletal concerns	12	3.14
Elevated lipids	7	2.33
Thyroid disorders	5	2.67
Circulation concerns	4	3.83
Mental health concerns	3	3.33

Focus Groups: Exploring Experiences and Strategies

The screening survey sample was used as a sampling frame to select members for focus groups to explore the range of experiences and strategies that these older adults employed to get through daily life while having multiple chronic conditions. Capitalizing on controlled group dynamics, focus group methodology is particularly well suited for exploratory studies and for generating ideas about habit-ridden topics (Krueger, 1998a, 1998b; Morgan, 1997, 1998a, 1998b). This qualitative research technique provided us with an understanding of the nature of the phenomenon of living with comorbidity from the older adults' perspective.

Sampling

Techniques of purposive sampling, with an emphasis on experiential compatibility, were used under the guiding principles of appropriateness and adequacy (Morse & Field, 1995). Appropriateness refers to the identification and selection of participants who could best inform the research. Adequacy refers to the quantity and quality of the data produced. Careful consideration of each of these principles minimizes sampling errors that threaten the validity of qualitative findings.

In consultation with David Morgan, a well-known expert on the use of focus groups in qualitative research, in November 1999, we decided that maximal variation within-group would best meet the research goals of this exploratory study. Therefore, in order to promote appropriateness of the data, the focus groups were segmented to establish compatibility (that is, to establish a sense of commonality among each groups' members) while maximizing variation within each group. The primary characteristics that drove segmentation were the number of reported conditions and the mean impact rating across these conditions. The number of conditions and impact were each segmented into three levels (high, moderate, low); then these levels were combined into nine iterations ranging from a *high* number of conditions with a *low* impact rating through a *low* number of conditions with *high* impact rating. Secondary characteristics included age and gender. For the purposes of this study, age was segmented at three levels: young-old (aged 55–64 years), middle-old (aged 65–74 years), and old-old (aged 75 and older). Gender was mixed to include at least two men per group to ensure some degree of compatibility.

Adequacy was addressed in consideration of group size and the number of groups planned. Three concerns guided decisions related to group size: the degree of participant involvement with the topic, the number of planned questions, and the desired length of the group discussion. Typically, focus groups have 6 to 10 participants per group; however, there is limited literature suggesting that age and impaired health status may influence these design considerations (Quine &

Cameron, 1995). Given the exploratory nature of the study, adequacy was addressed by planning a minimum of three groups, with continuation dependent on the degree of saturation achieved in the data (see Morgan, 1998b, for related focus group methodology, and Glaser & Strauss, 1967, for a discussion of principles of saturation.) Further, the use of a discussion guide enhanced the adequacy of data across groups.

The final sample derived for the focus group study included 37 older adults in five groups. Group size varied from 6 to 11 per group, with representation from each level of segmentation in terms of number of conditions, impact ratings, and age. At least two men attended each group, one who came with his wife and one who came alone. Thus, the segmentation plan was effectively applied to generate five groups that maximized variation within each theoretical segment.

Focus Group Format

The length of the sessions averaged 15 minutes for welcoming and organizing the group and 90 minutes for group interactions, followed by 15 minutes for thanking the participants and sharing in light refreshments. No group extended beyond a 2-hour time frame, out of respect for the participants who were volunteering their time. The group sessions were structured using Morgan's (1998b) "funnel design" and following the principles outlined by Krueger (1998b).

This approach to guided discussion flowed from introductory comments into broad general questions designed to facilitate compatibility, then into progressively more focused questions regarding how comorbidity affected daily life and what strategies were employed to manage these conditions. Summary activities included a round-table approach to rating the *most important* strategy for managing life with chronic conditions. This degree of structure was carefully designed to facilitate both content and thematic analysis of the data. (See Morse & Field, 1995, for general comments on analytic techniques; Krueger, 1998a, for focus group application.)

Moderation of the groups was also carefully addressed procedurally. A designated moderator led each group and was assisted by a co-moderator. The roles of the moderator and co-moderator were defined and discussed among the research team members to ensure consistency in roles. Moderators were trained to guide and focus the discussion, using probes to focus the inquiry without posing leading questions, while attending to time constraints and the flow of the discussion. Co-moderators served a supportive role, for example, attending to recording equipment and recording brief field notes of significant observations. Both the moderator and co-moderator participated in dictating debriefing notes, a form of field notes, following each session.

Data

Group interactions were recorded on audiotape and transcribed verbatim. First names were used to designate speakers in the transcription. Each tape was transcribed by an independent contractor, then verified by the moderator by listening to the tape while following the transcript word by word. This method minimized threats to validity posed by inaccurate transcription of spoken words, utterances, or emotional tones. In the process of verification, all identifiable referents were removed and replaced by a generic referent in brackets (for example, "Dr. Jones" was replaced by "Dr. [internist])." These verified transcripts were considered "clean," that is, confidentiality was protected and the data were prepared for further analysis. Thus, the primary data set consisted of clean transcripts and field notes generated after each group. In addition, each researcher maintained a log of key insights, and all analytic meetings were recorded for inclusion in the final data set.

Analytic Techniques

Both within-group and across-group analytic techniques were employed. Analysis started during group sessions as the participants related their life experiences. The process continued through listening to the audiotapes and through verification processes. All team members[1] received full sets (electronic files and printed copies) of clean transcripts for analysis. Team meetings with analytic and methodological foci were conducted at least weekly during the project to maximize the multiple perspectives afforded by working as a research team.

Two analytic techniques were employed: content analysis and thematic analysis. Content analysis refers to clusters such as information

---

[1]The full research team included the authors, two doctoral candidates in nursing, and three undergraduate summer scholars.

to develop taxonomies or lists that are all related to a common question or response. Thematic analysis draws more abstract theoretical threads from the data and provides conceptual insights into the process of living with multiple chronic illnesses. Morse and Field (1995) describe themes as "significant concepts that link substantial portions of the interviews together" (p. 140).

Working as a team, we conducted several analysis sessions focused on thematic analysis. Because the technique demands abstract, conceptual thinking, the most experienced qualitative researcher facilitated these sessions. The team was led through analysis of each group, identifying the conceptual threads in the data and then unifying these concepts into a model representing the process of living with multiple chronic conditions as illustrated by these older adults. A systematic process of verification or a challenge of the model using evidence provided in the data set was implemented to keep this analysis grounded in the experiential reality of the participants.

Then, using techniques of content analysis, the detailed responses of the participants were analyzed to flesh out the conceptual components of the model. For this type of analysis, the data were fractured by a question or response set, to detail the range of responses offered by the participants. This technique enabled the derivation of a categorical schema, for example, of the reported changes in daily life or of discrete strategies that these adults reported as part of their experience of living with multiple chronic illnesses.

Group Dynamics

Focus group methods are relatively dependent upon the interactions among group members and the moderators. These participants were eager to relate their experiences and discussed issues freely within the group sessions. Several of the older adults in each group were acquainted with one another through program or community activities; however, not all group members knew one another. Familiarity enhanced the group interactions as some members prompted others to relate an experience that they thought illustrated a point. There was no overt nonverbal or linguistic evidence that such interactions were uncomfortable for any of the members of the groups. It appeared that they had had such conversations regarding their health states before and were uninhibited in sharing their insights in a group forum.

Moderators used the discussion guide to maintain the group's focus on the topics of interest. Conversation flowed easily in the group settings, and all members contributed with minimal prompting. Overall, participants were courteous and respectful of fellow group members as they spoke. Even in times of divergent thinking, participants listened and then responded in turn, to disagree, extend, or illustrate a point. Affective responses, ranging from joking to crying, were manifest in each group. The largest group ($n = 11$ participants) was most difficult to keep focused, as group size seemed to influence the incidence of side conversations; thus, more frequent redirection or refocusing of the group was necessary.

Findings: Concerns of Comorbidity

Although health care practitioners, particularly physicians and advanced practice nurses, are taught to focus systemically on specific diagnoses, these older adults focused on seven broad areas of concern that transcend any particular chronic condition. Despite variation in the types and numbers of conditions experienced, age, and the overall health status of these older adults, their concerns overwhelmingly centered around energy, activity, sleep, diet, medication, attitudes, perceptions of self (sometimes as reflected by others), and additional sources of stress. Multiple diagnoses were cited in reference to these concerns, but the important finding was that the older adults thought holistically about their health rather than along diagnostic pathways for each condition. This, we believe, is the essence of comorbidity—living with multiple conditions that ultimately affect one's way of life in complex patterns that holistically supercede any one condition.

Issues surrounding energy included declining levels, conserving energy, avoiding depletion, and modifying practices. Overall, declining energy levels were reported as a primary concern that had ripple effects in other areas of life despite efforts to manage health, activity, and sleep and rest patterns. Strategies to conserve energy, such as minimizing the number of time stairs were negotiated in a given day, were common. Activity was closely monitored to avoid depletion of energy, a condition that was perceived as a significant threat. Everyday life was tailored to plan and modify practices with respect to threats to energy levels. For example, women spoke of a modified routine of cleaning one room at a time rather than tackling the whole house in one day, and men discussed extending household chores over days rather than hours.

With activity issues the focus was on ways used to adapt to the physical demands of daily life so that a desired daily routine could be maintained. It is important to keep in mind that these older adults were active, engaged people. They were proud to detail their schedules of events and heralded their contributions to family and community. But these activities were paced, energy was monitored throughout, and restrictions imposed by their conditions were minimized or controlled through treatment regimens or assistive devices.

The participants reported that their sleep was often disrupted by difficulties in falling asleep and frequent awakenings. Pain was a primary factor influencing sleep patterns, but early awakenings and difficulty getting to sleep without experiencing any pain were also common. For many, this time was used productively after several unsuccessful strategies to get to sleep. Some got out of bed to read, do craft projects, or even housecleaning chores to occupy their time less stressfully. Few participants reported worrying over sleeplessness; it was a phenomenon that was accepted as a natural part of aging and chronicity.

These older adults also universally discussed dietary restrictions as a major concern. Their dietary restrictions were complex and related to their multiple conditions. For many, a life adaptation incorporating one form of dietary restriction was later compounded by other restrictions. These lifestyle changes, for example, "not being able to eat what I want to," punctuated daily living and prompted "cheating" episodes when foods not recommended or prohibited were sought primarily for pleasure.

Medication routines marked the hours of each day with reminders of the conditions that these older folks endured. Though no specific information about medications taken by each participant was sought at any time during the study, each group raised concerns about medication. Some of these concerns are those commonly considered by practitioners, for example, cost and schedules. But other comments about taking medications revealed a more holistic concern: taking medication prolonged life and minimized symptoms, but medications for these types of conditions were *forever*. The adults' medication regimens primarily seemed to remind them of the existence of multiple conditions, pervading any sense of well-being with frequent reminders of their health concerns.

In the face of managing these multiple challenges in daily life, these adults felt aware of their conditions and reported changes in their attitudes and perceptions of self. They described how their lives had changed with the cumulative effects of multiple conditions. Strategies of self-comparison were frequently used as a bench mark of their own progress or decline and to minimize the perceived detrimental effects of their chronicity. Participants compared themselves to others of the same age, to those older, and even to those younger than they in an effort to gauge their own health status. Frequently, participants commented, "I'm doing okay compared to other people my age," or "When I see how bad other people have it, I'm doing okay."

Additional sources of stress were also reported in each group. The two most prominent ones were the loss of a spouse and ongoing caregiving responsibilities (for parents, disabled children, and grandchildren). The loss of a spouse was described as a blow that upset whatever balance had been achieved, resulting in a cascade of negative health events and a difficult path toward recovering lost ground. Ongoing caregiving was more of a nagging stressor that was challenging to energy levels. Even after the placement of older-adult loved ones into long-term-care facilities, the stress of caregiving drained precious energy and was carefully monitored in attempts to minimize the threat of energy depletion.

The Ecology of Coping with Comorbidity: Staying in Control

During the series of five focus group sessions, these elders told us in their own words what it is like to live with multiple health conditions. Chronic conditions had an impact on daily life in ways we had considered and also in other, more subtle ways. Unlike dealing with one condition, comorbidity presented a complex interplay of risk factors, symptoms, and treatment regimens. These older adults had learned to interpret, and in most cases respond effectively to, the complexity of managing their health in the face of chronicity.

They managed their lives, despite these conditions, through a dynamic flow of reading the scene, responding, and evaluating it, in an attempt to stay in control of conditions that threatened to dramatically impair their overall state of health. Many participants used combat analogies to describe this process. They likened it to "fighting a battle" or "waging a war" to control of their health so that they could perform desired daily activities. The model displayed in Figure 9.1 represents the process used by these adults to *stay in control* of the multiple conditions that threatened their ability to carry on. Each component of the

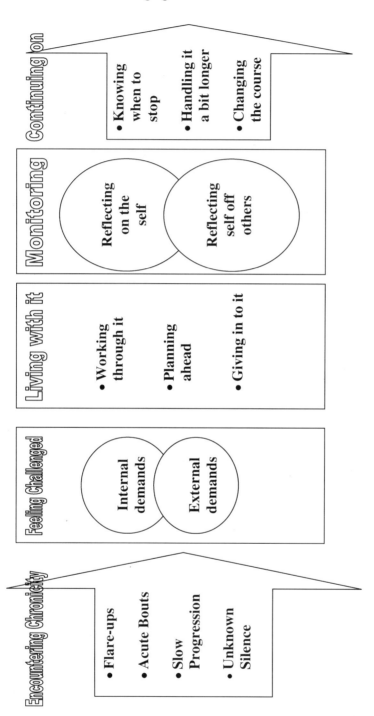

Figure 9.1 Living with multiple chronic conditions: staying in control.

model is illustrated and discussed separately; however, it is important to recall that these are dynamic interactions, not a linear stepwise flow.

Encountering Chronicity

Something brings chronic illness to the fore, and the older adult encounters chronicity with the comorbidity. Four modes of encountering were reported: flare-ups, slow progression, acute bouts, and unknowing silence.

Flare-Ups

These short-term exacerbations came and went, sometimes with discernable precursors, other times without warning. This mode was most common among those with arthritis and foot pain. For example, a 79–year-old woman with four chronic conditions reported

> My arthritis has a lot to do with this weather [rainy]. Isn't that funny? I can tell, I was saying to him [husband] earlier, I think we're going to have a good day 'cause that little constant pain is not there. And when it's going to be like this *dampness,* then I feel it.

A male participant in another group concurred. "In this kind of weather, I can become very stiff. It can be difficult for getting up and moving." Flare-ups presented a threat to the older adults because they were somewhat unpredictable, especially with conditions such as asthma. They tried to learn to predict the flare-ups and to be prepared to react, if necessary.

Slow Progression

For many, encountering chronicity meant facing a slow (often debilitating) progression of their conditions. This type of encounter was highlighted as participants described cumulative changes over time—for example, declining vision as cataracts matured prior to surgery, or degenerative joint disease that would eventually require joint replacement surgery. While they experienced no acute bouts, or even significant flare-ups, chronic conditions took their toll over time and culminated in noticeable declines. An 87–year-old man who reported five chronic conditions with a moderate impact score described his encounter with the slow progression of cataracts.

I would say the best part of a year that you're struggling along trying to read, and you can't read right. And you know I'd say it's a year. But there were six months between my first eye, the right, and they wouldn't do them both at one time. . . . It come on gradually. You don't realize what's the matter, and you start not being able to see, you know.

Acute Bouts

Sudden acute incidents punctuated the journey of living with chronicity. An 88–year-old man who was managing seven chronic conditions with a high-mean impact rating took an unfortunate fall that resulted in fracture, compounding his efforts to get by with his other conditions.

A year ago, I fell and broke my hip and what made me so sad was when I asked the doctor how the hip was, he said it was perfect. He didn't have to put [in] a new, uh, socket, just a new ball. I have no rheumatism or arthritis in that hip, and that's a shame. I wasted a good hip on that fall.

Others spoke of major medical events, such as urgent open-heart surgery, as an acute bout of a chronic condition within a much more extended flow of events, not as an isolated event. For example, one man spoke of his cardiac bypass surgery as part of his heart condition, but focused on how the surgery affected a long-term problem that he had with his leg following an automobile accident in early adulthood.

I favored that leg [the one injured in the auto accident], and after I had my heart surgery, my bad leg became my *good* leg because the other leg, it was so hard learning, like you learn a whole new lifestyle. Like I went up steps and I always put the good foot forth and bring up the other one. And you learn that. And for 12 years I had a system, and now that system was changed, and I was putting more stress on my bad leg. So now I have two *medium* legs.

Unknowing Silence

This mode describes how the older adults encountered conditions for which they were unable to assess or feel the effects. These conditions were described as "potentials," working into the elders' perspective of what the future might hold for them. This was a difficult mode to endure, especially because the silence provided no cues about whether their efforts to avoid serious consequences were effective. A 74-year-old woman discussed the silence of osteoporosis.

> I've been taking Fosamax for about three years. The first year, it seemed like there was an increase in the bone density. The next year, it was barely noticeable. So now I have to wait two years to have another bone density test. So I wonder to myself, "Why am I taking this Fosamax?" But maybe if I didn't, I'd be worse. I don't know.

Other conditions that were silent, not presenting symptomatic reminders, were risk factors such as family history for stroke or dementia, or altered lab values that were monitored periodically by the health care provider. Diabetes and hypertension were not described as silent because self-monitoring techniques provided evidence that was interpreted as a flare-up (e.g., one high reading), slow progression (e.g., stable readings), or an acute bout (e.g., serial high readings).

Feeling Challenged

The self-report of conditions that opened each focus group discussion revealed an important linguistic cue regarding feeling challenged. Typically prefaced by "I have [list of conditions]," participants often went on to say, "but my *problem* is . . . ." Having a "problem" differentiated the challenges of living with multiple chronic conditions. Though some conditions remained quietly under the surface, others rose to become a challenge in daily life. Challenges were based on both internal demands (e.g., dealing with pain) and external demands (e.g., walking up steps to get to the bathroom) on the person. Feeling challenged represents the ways that chronicity had an impact on the lives of these elders as they sensed these demands throughout the flow of everyday life.

Internal Challenges

Intra-individual demands were sensed as these older adults went about daily life. Their bodies posed internal challenges as they worked to manage a daily routine. Internal challenges were categorized around limitations in movement, pain, or discomfort; declining energy levels, poor sleep, and dietary restrictions. Though many of these were physical challenges, the participants described an affective component as well, such as "It messes with my mind."

External Challenges

Numerous environmental demands are placed on the older person at home and in other settings. For example, one 71–year-old woman with movement limitations described how the location of the sink in her home created a challenge for her. "Because of my space I don't have an upstairs bathroom, so I have to carry my water from the kitchen up." Steps presented a special challenge, especially during flare-ups: "Well . . . some days, . . . going up steps is very difficult. . . . And there's some days like it's not worth the effort to go up." Others described the challenges posed by parking and traffic at local shopping centers: "You don't mind when you could get in the door, you don't mind it until you leave, but the parking and the getting to and from the stores is a problem." Therefore, environmental challenges abound, both in the home and in the community.

Living with It

"You just gotta live with it" was a phrase commonly used by these older adults. In order to "live with it," they employed a variety of coping strategies. The use and selection of strategies were very dynamic, that is, the older adults changed strategies or moved between the styles of "living with it" in response to ever-changing challenges. While they relied on past successes for determining what to do in the present, these adults creatively adapted new strategies in response to the challenges presented them. As described by an active 71–year-old, "You have to be ready to switch gears very quickly."

Several discrete strategies were used as forms of coping with chronic conditions or to manage particular concerns through living with them. The most prevalent strategies included taking medications, exercising, changing dietary patterns, seeking information, practicing religion, and keeping busy. These strategies were used across three primary modes of "living with it": working through it, planning ahead, or giving in to it.

Working Through It

Working through it was the most common style of living with it, as the older adult responsively accommodated the challenges set forth in daily life. Participants described this process as "just keep on keeping on." Many worked through discomfort in this mode, but did not want to "give in to it." As one woman explained, "Some days it's not worth the effort. But then, that's giving in to it, so you reverse your thinking and you go about your business each day."

Planning Ahead

Though working through it was a form of responsive coping, planning ahead was proactive coping. These adults would implement strategies to block the detrimental effects of the chronic conditions from interfering with their activities so that they could do more in a given day. One respondent aptly described these types of activities as "protecting yourself."

A common form of planning ahead involved pacing movement or activities to preserve energy. As one participant humorously put it,

> When I bend over to tie my shoes, I look around to see if there's anything else I can do while I'm [down] there. I sort of do that in everything. . . . You just make slight adjustments all around to get away from more exertion.

Planning ahead takes both challenges and demands into consideration. For example, for those with the urgency and frequency of diuretic needs or prostate disorders, knowing where public restrooms were located became a prime concern. One man casually commented,

> Another thing people want to know, most of them, is where the restrooms are . . . That's one of the first things you find out, which is in your head—do they have a rest room *here*? Do they have a restroom *there*? That's a big item.

Others echoed this concern, discussing personal situations in which they were planning ahead by checking the environment for resources to manage their needs.

Giving In to It

While waging a battle against the ravages of multiple chronic conditions, there were times when a person just couldn't fight any longer. Participants reported feeling overwhelmed, depressed, or as if they "just can't do it" and so give in. Some strategies that were used when giving in included lying down, medicating, or relinquishing the day's activities.

Although some strongly fought against giving in, others used it as a form of taking a break. For example, some gave in until their medication kicked in to diminish the pain that kept them from completing their activities. In a few cases, giving in was a protracted period that was much more difficult to break. One woman related her story of giving in to arthritis: "I didn't walk for 10 months, it was so bad." She has subsequently worked her way through it, resumed her walking program, and now suffers only occasional flare-ups.

Monitoring

Throughout these dynamics of feeling challenged and responding by living with it, the participants universally discussed two types of monitoring activities. They used the technique of reflecting introspectively on their self, to assess their current state in comparison to a baseline or their own expectation. In addition, they often reflected in relation to others as they reframed their image of health based on interactions with others. These monitoring activities appeared to be balanced because they listened to their bodies to assess their state of health, compared themselves to others, and carefully presented an outward picture of their state of health to others in their social network.

Reflecting on the Self

Using this monitoring activity, the participants focused on listening to their bodies. A form of short-term assessment, reflecting on one's self most often revolved around challenges that they had experienced: Had they escalated, resolved, or stayed about the same? Reflecting on the self cued the individual to changes in demand (either internal or external), thus allowing for changes in expectations for achievement. For some, this meant doing more, for example, cutting the grass while a pain pill was maximally effective. For others, demands increased or energy was depleted, calling for a lowering of expectations for the day: I always make a list of what I want to do, and I used to get real frustrated when I didn't get the whole list done . . . There were times when my illness, I feel frustrated, but I don't feel well enough to get everything done. But I've learned . . . that the housework is going to be there tomorrow . . . So instead of looking at this list and thinking,

Boy, I have five more things and I didn't get them done, I look at the four things and am glad I got *them* done

Reflecting Off Others

While reflecting on the self was an introspective assessment, but reflecting on one's self by comparison with others indicated how older adults reframed their images of self through these interactions with others. Self-comparison and maintaining an image of health were commonly discussed in the focus groups. Social networks provided the means for reflecting off others.

Comparing one's state of health to that of others was described frequently, often as part of the introductions early in the focus groups. Despite reporting 10 chronic conditions (some of which, from a medical perspective, would be considered life-threatening), one man commented, "I feel blessed listening to everybody else." Volunteer work often exposed the participants to others who were considered "worse off," forming a regular basis for self-comparison. A 79–year-old woman who worked as a hospital volunteer and reported having three chronic conditions with a high impact rating, noted, "I see some awful sights, and I figure I'm real lucky in what I can do. I'm really lucky." Interestingly, this comparison was not only limited to people of the same or similar age, but also to those who were perceived to be significantly older or younger than they.

Overall, self-comparison produced positive feelings of being lucky, blessed, or thankful. At times, self-comparison was a stimulus to perform, in a competitive fashion.

> Like, when I walk . . . I'll walk, and then somebody comes older than me. And boy, they go hightailing, and I can never catch them. Like this one lady, I knew she would never make it around the track the second time, and she was walking slow, and I thought good, I finally beat somebody. And by God, she passed me. The pass was a warm-up.

An 81-year-old man who was plagued with chronic pain, described how reflecting off of others stimulated him to walk, even through his pain.

> We walk every morning . . . I can't keep up with [my wife], but I walk with friends and they walk faster than I would normally like to, and I have to keep up, and that's good for me. That helps me push myself in

the morning. And I hurt, I really hurt. But I force myself to go, and handle it.

Only one woman differed on positive outcomes through self-comparison, finding it difficult to accept changes in herself even when she perceived that she was better off than others.

> It's just sometimes, then you stop and think, oh God, I'm really lucky, you know. Look at somebody else and you think, oh gosh. I *should* count my blessings, but sometimes. But I mean, like, I used to swim a mile when I went swimming. Now I'm lucky if I can do a little better than a quarter of a mile . . . and I think I've had a big day. It sort of makes you feel like, oh, what's happening to me.

Continuing On

Elaborating on their introspective processes of reflecting on the self and the more socially based self-reflection of comparison with others, these older adult participants described their continuation of the journey of living with multiple chronic conditions as following three pathways. The first was *knowing when to stop*. On this path, feedback was interpreted as serious or significant markers (termed by one participant as "cautions") that signaled a need to stop pushing onward. These were the signs of *overdoing*, a phenomenon that appeared to be relatively common among this group. They carefully assessed whether the origin of a pain in the neck was muscular strain or angina. Knowing when to stop exemplified how these elders used lessons from the past to read the present situation to avert serious problems. One woman reported feeling "awfully warm and sweaty" during exercise and had to rest, fearing that she was about to have another heart attack. Stopping was not an easy way out of the constant battle; it was a resignation to heeded cautions discovered in reflecting on the self.

When the feedback was not as ominous, the participants described *handling it a bit longer*. On this path, they pushed through discomforting or especially challenging situations to keep on the designated track toward their goals for performance. Handling it a bit longer was the predominant course, following monitoring. A woman in chronic pain described this pathway clearly: "I think that's the key to daily living. You have to rise above it, even though you don't want to, but you say, I can do this. And then you *do it*. But it doesn't mean you're in less pain, or you—it's just that you have to."

Changing course was the third pathway used, described as a significant change in how the older adults dealt with their multiple chronic conditions. Most of the participants described a responsive effort to deal with their conditions independently until they had adequate feedback or new information that indicated things just weren't right. Talking with the doctor was a major theme of changing the course. These adults felt a great personal responsibility for their health and a need to present their situation thoroughly and accurately. As the group nodded in agreement, one man summarized: "A lot of these things [strategies] you pick up, but the problem is you almost have to be a doctor yourself to get the right treatment. You almost have to guide them and say this is my problem." At times, the change in course focused on a treatment, for example, starting or discontinuing a medication. At other times, the change was more dramatic. When participants felt that their doctors were not listening or responding aptly to their situation, they persevered in changing the course by having a "straight talk" with the doctor, by reiterating a need, or even by finding a new provider.

Staying in Control

As the older adult lives with multiple chronic conditions, this trajectory becomes reiterative with movement through the conceptual components of the model within the dynamic flow of everyday life. Most of the strategies used to deal with comorbidity in everyday life were described as a quest to "just keep what I have." When not in a period of accruing significant losses, maintaining the current baseline state of health was the predominant concern. Looking retrospectively at their situations, the older adults in the focus groups related periods of gaining, losing, and maintaining capabilities in their personal history of living with multiple chronic conditions.

Gains were almost universally presented as the fruits of their labors in overcoming the disabling consequences of comorbidity. These small incremental changes marked a degree of success for these older adults. Exercise was most illustrative, as one woman reported,

> I'm getting up and down better. In church I used to have to get a hold of the front pew to pull myself up. Now I get up with my head up and no problem. And there are many things. I can stoop better now.

Small incremental gains were related to personal behaviors, but more significant gains were often attributed to surgery (especially cardiac bypass surgery) that resulted in a markedly changed capability to go through life with more energy and a new lease on life.

Although some losses were sudden, such as those that occurred with an injury or acute illness, slow progressive losses were expected as a part of aging. Participants would frequently attribute their chronicities to aging, by saying things like, ". . . arthritis, which I think comes with age for all of us." Another participant related expectations for losses with aging by saying, "It's frustrating really, when you stop to think about it. Then you think, well, I'm lucky. Then you think, well, the older you get the worse it's going to get."

Implications

Our preliminary model of Staying in Control is conceptually congruent with extant theory on coping. This new model is differentiated from previous work by its focus on the process of coping with multiple chronic conditions. This shift toward understanding coping with more than two conditions that interplay in a complex fashion is important because comorbidity is a way of life for most older adults.

This study addressed coping from a broad theoretical perspective that encompassed all actions, thoughts, or feelings that contributed to the older adults' management of multiple chronic conditions. We never used the term "coping" in our discussion groups, to avoid issues surrounding the scope of the term (as described by Bennett, Weinman, & Spurgeon, 1990); however, at least one older adult in each group used that word to describe their living with multiple chronic illnesses.

Lazarus and Folkman's (1984) work in the field of stress and coping is perhaps the most common model employed for understanding coping responses. According to their model, an appraisal of threat is the first phase of a coping response. Because comorbidity is so complex, there are two conceptually distinct elements in the appraisal phases identified in the Staying in Control model. First, in encountering chronicity the older adults described how they were aware that their conditions would be with them for life; their illnesses would not go away or be cured. The major dimensions of how one perceives illness described by Scharloo et al. (1998) and Lipowski (1970) were evident in this appraisal phase; however, this study did not reveal patterns of coping driven by these perceptions of illness.

Given this baseline appraisal of the multiple factors on the horizon of their existence, facing challenges in daily life presented a more specific appraisal of the demands or challenges rooted in the person (i.e., body, mind, and spirit) and contextual challenges they faced at that time or on that day. The four functions of coping described by Pearlin and Schooler (1978) were evidenced in the older adults' discussion of how they handled these challenges. They talked about keeping their stress levels down, of changing how they reframed things that they just could not change, about using religion and spirituality to establish new meaning for their altered lives as they aged with multiple conditions, and certainly about managing symptoms and challenges presented by their conditions.

The more traditional models of coping feature some form of reappraisal. For example, Lazarus and Folkman (1984) describe how reappraisal that occurs during the process of determining strategies may create a feedback that changes the perception of the threat. In the Staying in Control model, reappraisal emerged as a distinct phase of the process called "checking on myself." A unique contribution of our work is the identification of the internal and external processes of reflection that these older adults used in reappraisal of their situations. On the topic of "reflecting on myself," they specifically discussed an introspective attitude of "listening to the body" as a form of reappraisal. In addition, the process of reflecting on their self in relation to others makes social support networks a source for gaining insights on others' perceptions of their state of health and for projecting a controlled image of their own health. Based on these assessments, the older adults in this study described three patterns of continuing on (i.e., knowing when to stop, handling it a bit longer, and changing course)—all representing advancement through the process rather than reverting to earlier phases.

The Folkman and Lazarus (1984) model described a negative emotion that leads to an appraisal of threat or harm, yet the older adults in our study did not seem to perceive the challenges of daily life as particularly threatening or necessarily harmful. Rather, they described being challenged as "just the way it is." Living with comorbidity becomes a way of life for these adults and includes a dynamic flow of patterned accommodations (manifested in the coping phases "living with it," "checking on myself," and "continuing on"). The only phase of the Staying in Control model derived from this sample that addresses perception of a threat or harm is *knowing when to stop*. This is a unique method of coping whereby older adults pause or stop, heeding serious or ominous warning signals that prompt them to alter their course begin to sense they have pushed too hard.

Although the literature on coping describes both discrete strategies and styles that are developed over time, we found a more dynamic flow of patterned responses that blended multiple strategies toward a goal (i.e., giving in, working through it, or planning ahead). These older adults often mentioned discrete strategies, yet they were framed in the patterns of living with it, checking on myself, and continuing on. These patterns are not the same as coping styles that are based on individual characteristics. They are patterned "styles" that are based on, and perhaps have evolved from, the experience of comorbidity. We expect that individual coping styles may present different manifestations within each pattern—that is, how the older adult chooses and mixes strategies to persist in life, when succumbing would most likely be the more traditional style of personal coping.

Finally, a key element of the Lazarus and Folkman work (1984) is their emphasis on an assessment of effectiveness and expectations for the future. We learned important lessons from these elders that shed light on these assessments. The effectiveness of a strategy becomes more complicated in chronic comorbidity. What are the measures of effectiveness? From the perspective of the older adults in this study, the answer is equivocal.

Their first level of assessment of effectiveness was in "checking on myself" as they monitored their bodies for clues that their current course of action was effective in meeting the challenges of daily life. But on a higher level, the adults carefully monitored the course of their conditions: Were they holding them in check? Were they progressing despite their efforts? A higher level of effectiveness was thus of concern to them. Living with chronicity is a lifelong event, so assessing the effectiveness of coping has become a more protracted assessment that permeates the day-to-day lives of these elders.

As we listened to these people tell their stories of living with two or more chronic conditions, we began to wonder about the appropriateness of their courses of action. When is "giving in" a health-promoting course of action, and when does it become detrimental to long-term health? If the older adult is happy with the selected course but is misreading cues, is this effective? Roth and Cohen (1986) assert that in the face of a situation deemed uncontrollable, denial may actually be the most effective strategy. Given the contextual factors of the lifelong journey of living with chronic conditions, such strategies may be effective but not the most beneficial for the older adult. This is another key contribution of this work: though a particular course or strategy may be effective in confronting a challenge, it may not be the most efficacious for maximizing the older adult's health over time.

White, Richter, and Fry (1992) broach the idea of appropriateness in their study, demonstrating that overreliance on escape-avoidance or wishful thinking relates to poor adjustment to diabetes. These strategies may have reduced the stress of being diabetic, but they were not very effective in successfully managing this potentially life-threatening condition. In future studies, an external assessment using established criteria of appropriateness might augment our understanding of the effectiveness of coping from the perspective of long-term health promotion rather than from immediate stress response.

Typically, coping responses are categorized according to three higher-order constructs: problem-based coping that focuses on managing external aspects of the stressor; emotion-focused or cognitive strategies that regulate internal or emotional reactions to the stressor; and avoidance. Though the strategies identified in this study fit this framework, their true constructed meanings were not evident in our discussions with these older adults. The dynamic flow and blended patterns of strategies identified in the model of Staying in Control more accurately represent the reality of these older adults' experiences with daily life. If this model holds among other samples, it may provide important insights for understanding how professional intervention may alter this course (if needed) to obtain even higher levels of health and wellness. Furthermore, we must understand the perspectives of older adults to enable effective communication within a framework that makes sense to them. Thus, constructs developed for scientific investigation are inadequate for this purpose.

Our emphasis on Staying in Control was rooted in the older adults' accounts of daily lives that are fraught with the challenges posed by as many as 11 chronic conditions. They fought hard battles, using a full range of coping responses to maintain a sense of being in control of their conditions, even if that meant consciously deciding to "give in" for a while. These findings are not consistent with Keller's (1988) assertion that perceptions of control or manageability are related to the types of strategies one chooses; yet it is important to recall that this sample was purposively selected to allow us to study older adults who were managing well enough to live independently in the community and to attend social and educational programming events. Further study is needed to explore the experience of comorbidity among home-bound and institutionalized older adults and other independent older adults who are not managing chronicity well enough to engage in community programming. Such studies may reveal alternative perceptions of control and, subsequently, coping pathways among other samples.

Conclusions

In conclusion, it is comforting to know that the extant theory on coping was well supported by this study of older adults with multiple chronic conditions. We have gained new insights regarding how older adults who are coping effectively may feel challenged but not threatened as they implement self-care strategies in everyday life. We have identified the blended coping strategies that older adults have used in response to these challenges. We have raised the issues of appropriateness of selected courses of coping to promote long-term health and well-being. And, we have integrated the reflective processes of introspection and reflection, with projection within a social network, as forms of monitoring or appraisal used by these adults. These insights provide fertile ground for continued study of how older adults use effective and appropriate coping responses not only to resolve the stressors of their multiple chronic conditions but also to maximize their capabilities in order to achieve a state of health and well-being.

Though this study has shed important insights on how older adults live with multiple chronic conditions, we have only scratched the surface of this complex life circumstance. This exploratory research was constrained by necessary sampling and methodological design decisions. It is crucial to move this line of research even closer to the lived experience of the individual, for example, through daily process research techniques. Continued study of other similar and different samples is necessary to discern commonalities and divergence in the experience of living with comorbidity. Through further research we hope to unravel the complexities of comorbidity to enable interventions that maximize capability in the face of potentially disabling conditions.

Chapter 10

Coping with Multiple Chronic Health Conditions

Peter Martin

C hronic diseases are now responsible for 80% of all deaths in Western societies (McKinlay & McKinlay, 1977). With increasing life expectancy, most older adults can expect to live with at least one chronic disease during the later part of their lives. As Maes, Leventhal, and de Ridder (1996) point out, there is no single, universally accepted medical definition of chronic illness because there are important differences in the causes, course, changeability, and consequences of chronic conditions. Usually the focus is on chronic conditions that are most prevalent, have a major impact on the health care system, or that have a high rate of mortality.

As older adults learn to live with chronic conditions, even with multiple chronic conditions, they are challenged to find effective ways of coping with chronic diseases. *Coping* is typically considered a generic term summarizing all thoughts and behaviors in reaction to stressful situations (Lazarus, 1986). As a generally stabilizing factor, coping can help individuals maintain psychosocial adaptation during stressful periods (Holohan, Moos, & Schaefer, 1996). The basic assumption in stress and coping models is that people are confronted with a stressor (e.g., a chronic disease), appraise the stressor, and with that appraisal, determine a coping response (Lazarus & Folkman, 1984). In many cases, the coping response that is chosen is thought to predict different levels of adjustment.

Response to Previous Articles

For individuals with multiple chronic diseases, coping becomes the key to effective adaptation.[1] The papers by Poon, Basford, Dowzer, and Booth; Basford; Poon, Dowzer, and Booth; and Penrod, Gueldner, and Poon that comprise the three preceding chapters all focus on coping, primarily with regard to chronic health conditions.

The following sections of this chapter raise three primary questions in response to these articles: First, what role do patterns of multiple chronic conditions play when considering coping responses and successful adaptation? Second, what conceptual issues need to be addressed? And third, what are effective coping responses in reaction to chronic conditions?

This review ends with several suggestions for future work. In the endnotes to this chapter, we provide additional salient points made by several participants at the AARP Andrus Foundation invitational conference held in February 2002 in San Francisco, where the papers were first presented and discussed.

What Role Do Patterns of Multiple Chronic Conditions Play?

Poon, Basford, Dowzer, and Booth (chapter 7) cite Feinstein's (1970) definition of comorbidity, "an associated illness arising from other diseases," and the somewhat broader definition, namely, the coexistence of three types of diseases. Comorbidity does not necessarily imply chronic conditions, however. For example, an individual might have arthritis (typically considered to be a chronic condition), but at the same time may be having an acute bout with the common cold. This combination of acute and chronic diseases would be different from someone who has two chronic diseases, such as arthritis and cancer.

Chronic diseases may also interact with other stressful events that are not health-related. Consider, for example, a person who has diabetes. The disease may be quite manageable until this person experiences a divorce or mourns the death of a spouse. With this additional

---

[1]Robert Kahn reminded us that the coping literature is focused largely on specific episodes, such as bereavement, victimization, accidents, or illness. Taking an episode-driven notion about coping and applying to chronic diseases is a challenging task. Just as the event literature has begun to distinguish between different types of events (hassles, personal events, historical events), the coping literature might need to find ways to define behaviors in response to different chronic diseases.

stressful event, established coping patterns may be severely compromised.

These examples demonstrate that it is important to keep clarity about the patterns of multiple chronic conditions before considering coping responses and successful adaptation. Rather than counting up the number of stressful events (or diseases), as is often done in the stress and coping literature, researchers could contribute much to our understanding of coping with comorbidity by establishing patterns of disease management.

The review of the most common comorbidities provided by Basford et al. is a useful start to evaluate the relative importance of comorbidity patterns. For example, the health conditions of coronary heart disease and major depression link a physical with a mental disease, while the combination of congestive heart failure and diabetes links two major physical diseases. Effective coping responses are very likely to be different for persons with from these different disease patterns. An important contribution of research addressing comorbidity is that differential patterns can be ascertained.

Although there are few studies about coping with comorbidity, as Basford et al. note in chapter 8, some literature is available highlighting coping responses for specific diseases (Maes et al., 1996). For example, those who have asthma tend to minimize the problem and are typically self-confident about overcoming the disease (Woller et al., 1992). Patients who have cancer are known to use emotion-focused responses (de Ridder & Schreurs, 1994). The literature on coronary heart disease suggests that denial is common at least as an initial response to the diagnosis (Gentry, Foster, & Haney, 1972). Finally, examples from diabetes research indicate that active responses and internal control are quite common for this disease (Frenzel, McCaul, Glasgow, & Schafer, 1988). Taken together, these examples suggest that there are great individual differences in the way that older adults deal with chronic diseases, depending on the prevailing disease. The comorbidity of diseases would call for even more differentiated results. Consider an adult who has asthma and diabetes. Would this person be more likely to be active, as suggested by the diabetes literature; or to minimize the importance of the chronic diseases, as suggested by the asthma literature? The most likely scenario would be for this individual to minimize one disease but become active in dealing with the other. The picture perhaps changes if this person perceives a new chronic disease as "just too much," and any secondary chronic disease, or perhaps the one that appears least threatening, is neglected. One disease may become the dominant one to deal with, a second or third may be neglected. Some individuals consequently may decide that they can only manage one disease at a time. Other individuals may be able to focus on multiple chronic diseases simultaneously.

A final issue concerns the role of the disease itself versus the symptoms shown by the disease. Are individuals coping with blood pressure problems or with the symptoms of dizziness? Are people with diabetes coping with the disease or with the restrictions in their diet? Coping may inform about relevant strategies of daily living rather than about disease management. When coping questions are addressed, general problems or events are typically considered as the triggers for coping. In the case of chronic diseases, however, it may be important whether individuals cope with the disease itself or with its symptoms.[2] The issues discussed so far suggest that more work needs to be done on the conceptual level. Our discussion therefore turns to the necessity for conceptual models.

What Conceptual Issues Need to Be Addressed?

Stress and coping models such as the one proposed by Penrod, Gueldner, and Poon in chapter 9 can inform us about differential pathways of coping with comorbidity. Assessing such pathways would be an important contribution to the stress and coping literature that typically is monolithic (one event) or global (a number of stressors encountered). One of the reasons for which the stress and coping research is in somewhat of a disarray, as pointed out by Poon et al. in chapter 7, may have to do with the fact that many different health conditions can serve as stimuli for general coping responses.

The model introduced by Penrod et al. is a useful heuristic start, informing us about important model elements to be considered in work with multiple chronic diseases. However, the process model is based on the authors' careful data collection and includes the "voices" of their study participants. This model is very appealing and may allow for the testing of different pathways. First, the direct pathway from

---

[2]Margaret Wallhagen pointed out that individuals suffering from multiple chronic diseases may also deal with "symptom confusion,"which often makes it difficult for individuals to respond effectively. For example, adults who have diabetes may complain about vision problems or fatigue, which may be blamed on usual aging. In these cases, aging symptoms, functional impairment, and symptoms of diabetes may be confusing to individuals.

chronic stress, through stress appraisals, to behavioral coping may be tested (see Figure 10.1). An alternative model would include dimensions of internal demands (see Figure 10.2), whereas a third model would focus on the inclusion of external demands as additional mediators (see Figure 10.3).

It should be noted that these models reflect an oversimplification of the much richer and more complex model developed by Penrod et al.(chapter 9). The suggested pathways of the Penrod model include chronic stress or combinations thereof as independent variables exerting an effect on external and internal demands. The demands as well as chronic stress are appraised or monitored, which in turn predicts coping responses. This model is quite testable, and chronic conditions could be viewed as a moderating variable, evaluating whether the model works equally well for different diseases or patterns of disease. For example, we may ask whether the link from chronic stress to internal demands to coping is the strongest part for one particular disease, whereas the link between chronic stress, external demands, and coping is more important for another disease. What are the predictive lines for someone who has high blood pressure? Perhaps the link between stress and internal demands is more pronounced for this subgroup, although stress is more likely to affect external demands for those who have had a stroke and are homebound. These demands might in turn affect appraisal processes leading to different modes of behavioral coping: the person with high-blood pressure may be more likely to engage in changes of health behavior (nutrition, exercise), while the person who has had a stroke may be more engaged in home modifications that allow for high levels of activity.

Additional variations of this "dynamic" model could include the severity or the impact of the chronic conditions as suggested by Penrod et al. Perceptions about the impact of chronic diseases add an important dimension.[3] A threshold model could also be evaluated: comparing those who score high or low on the severity for a chronic condition to show differential effects on coping. It could be hypothesized that individuals are more likely to drain reserve energy levels after a certain threshold is reached.

---

[3]Leonard Poon made the observation that metacognitions may be involved in the perception of chronic diseases. Some people may very consciously explicate their coping behaviors, while others may use coping behaviors without reflecting much on them or fully understanding the circumstances surrounding a disease and its resulting coping behaviors. In a similar vein, Vaillant (2000) introduced the terms "conscious cognitive strategies" and "involuntary mental mechanisms."

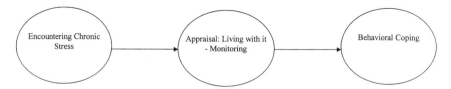

Figure 10.1 Hypothesized coping model: Chronic stress, appraisal, and coping.

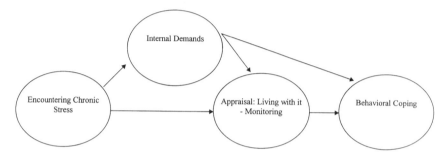

Figure 10.2 Hypothesized coping model: Chronic stress, internal demands, appraisal, and coping.

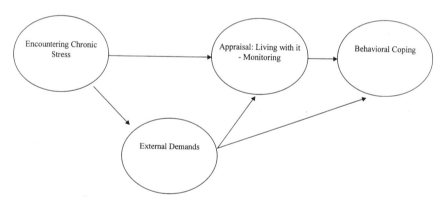

Figure 10.3 Hypothesized coping model: Chronic stress, external demands, appraisal, and coping.

Alternatively researchers may want to assess cumulative chronic stresses in the ways suggested by Basford et al. (chapter 8) and Lepore and Evans (1996): as additive effects, multiplicative effects, and main effects. Additive effects would increase adjustment problems in a linear way, while multiplicative effects would either attenuate or potentiate the effect of chronic stress, depending on the stressor. Main effects would simply indicate that two chronic diseases show independent effects on adjustment problems. Although this model serves to explain how older adults cope with multiple chronic conditions, the next important question is concerned with the evaluation of effective coping responses.

What Are Effective Coping Responses?

Basford et al. in chapter 8 remind us that coping responses differ, depending on the naturalistic framework, culture, expectations, and frequency of experience. But ultimately, individuals who have chronic diseases would like to know what works and what does not work. To cite Zeidner and Saklofske (1996), "Coping strategies work with modest effects, sometimes, with some people" (p. 520). It is therefore very difficult to establish any major guidelines or recommendations of effective coping responses. Pearlin and Schooler (1978) reminded us almost 25 years ago that specific coping responses are either more or less effective, depending on the type of stress encountered.

Rather than assessing general coping responses as effective or not, it may be more fruitful to ask whether individuals maintain a store of coping skills that they can draw from in any given situation. Effective coping would entail a larger repertoire of response possibilities and be more flexible, and different responses potentially could be combined to deal with a chronic disease (Strack & Feifel, 1996). A repertoire of coping also suggests that some general coping patterns are used across many situations, while some specific coping responses are used only in specific circumstances (Sperling, 2000). In essence, individuals coping with chronic diseases may already possess coping tools. In some situations, certain coping tools help with the chronic stress; in other situations, other tools may be helpful. For example, when arthritis flares up, perhaps taking pain medication is the best tool available; however, when individuals are diagnosed with a new disease, reading up on the problem (i.e., information seeking) may be the tool of choice. People who cope best and most effectively are perhaps able to find the right tool for the right symptom at the right time. When symptoms appear, individuals may first ask which tools are potentially available, which of those available tools they want to use, and what the consequences would be if a certain coping tool were used. Some tools may be available in almost any situation, while other tools are only available in very specific situations, but when these situations come up, it is very important to have these special tools available. Along the same line, some coping tools may be very helpful in some situations, but harmful in others.[4]

A particular coping response may differentially influence various outcomes (Silver & Wortman, 1980). Denial of a chronic condition may reduce emotional stress, but may compromise health care choices that would be utilized if the person were not using denial as the primary coping response (Strack & Feifel, 1996). Finally, it should be emphasized that coping adaptiveness may vary across phases of a stressful encounter. Active behavioral coping responses typically help in the detection of chronic diseases; denial, on the other hand, is an emotional response used to minimize the life-threatening aspects of a chronic disease. Timing is also important for adaptive coping. Though avoidance responses may be more effective for short-term stressors, active coping responses would be more beneficial for long-term stressors (Strack & Feifel, 1996; Suls & Fletcher, 1985).

From the Penrod et al. study, it is clear that cognitive coping mechanisms are just as important as behavioral ones: It appears to be important to work through important issues cognitively, reflecting on the situation and giving in when necessary. Individuals who have multiple chronic diseases may find themselves too challenged at times and decide that it is time to give in for the day. Maybe tomorrow there will be new opportunities to deal with the disease, but not today. If this is the case, as the Penrod et al. study suggests, then it would be important to undertake short-term longitudinal studies that allow for daily or weekly coping assessments.

A second useful mechanism for those with multiple chronic conditions appears to be responses of social comparison (i.e., what Penrod et al. call "reflecting off others"). To maintain successful levels of adaptation, older adults who have multiple chronic conditions may be compromised in their active coping response choices but continue to maximize and utilize cognitive modes of coping. This would be similar to the oldest-old who have also been reported to maintain relatively high levels of cognitive coping (Martin et al., 1992; Martin, Rott, Poon, Courtenay, & Lehr, 2001).[5]

---

[4]Margaret Wallhagen added an important question to our discussion: Why do people choose certain coping reactions over others? Why do they think that they would work?
[5]Margaret Wallhagen made the point that choices of coping may be limited by the situational dynamics and available resources in given situations.

Future Research Considerations

In this final section, I would like to point to some future directions of research, study, and application that can build on the work presented by Poon et al., Basford et al., and Penrod et al. in the earlier chapters. To some extent these thoughts and suggestions may also be relevant to other contributions to this book.

First, it seems that most stress and coping studies take a relatively narrow time frame when assessing successful adaptation. We have recently made the point that too few studies of adaptation include distal influences that help to explain why an individual successfully copes with adversity or not (Martin & Martin, 2002). A life-span view of adaptation would include important biographical or life history data, rather than just an assessment of the current chronic condition with its resulting coping responses. How well an individual copes with multiple chronic conditions may depend much more on past experiences and positive or negative relationships with others in the past. The "developmental adaptation" assessed over longer periods of time and in combination with individual and social resources may add significantly to our understanding of the stress and coping process in individuals who have multiple chronic conditions (Martin, in press).

Another timing issue relates to the question of age and duration. As Felton and Revenson (1987) point out, being old *and* having a serious illness may lead to less active, submissive, and somewhat more pessimistic means of coping. Furthermore, does it matter for how long individuals have had from a chronic disease? At what time did a second or third chronic disease enter the biographical picture? It seems that timing and duration have been neglected in most coping research but should be considered when chronicity of diseases is involved. Second, we should underline the question of whether some coping responses are universal (Poon et al., chapter 7) or habitual ("traits"), and others situational (Beehr & McGrath, 1996) or time-specific (Poon et al.). If some coping responses are useful or effective across situation and time, then they could be viewed as stable coping traits available in almost every stressful situation. Certain coping responses, on the other hand, may be very specific to the stressor encountered or the timing of a chronic condition. A differential view of coping that accounts for the combination of chronic diseases is in all likelihood more fruitful than assessing global scores of active or passive coping.

Further refinement of coping models is needed in future research. Although much attention has been paid to including salient proximal variables in stress and coping models, there has been much less attention to the time-relatedness within the process of stress and coping. How much time passes between the experience of chronic stressors until resources are mobilized, between the utilization of resources and coping responses to chronic stressors? Finally, how much time passes between coping and the benefits of coping? Obviously stress and coping models should be evaluated with prospective designs, but it seems equally important to pay attention to the importance of time intervals between predictors, mediators, and outcomes. When dealing with severe pain, shorter time units may be appropriate, while monitoring elevated blood pressure may require a longer time frame.

More work is also needed to develop disease-specific coping instruments (Maes et al., 1996). If coping is disease-specific, then we should not assume that the same coping measure is appropriate for all chronic diseases. A coping measure for arthritis may include more items that focus on self-monitoring techniques. A coping measure for cardiovascular disease may have an extended section on coping responses that include engagement in specific health behaviors.

Finally, Basford et al. (chapter 8) remind us that we should ask whether coping is and should be modifiable. Specific coping behaviors, such as exercising, seeking social support, and using nutritional behaviors, are all part of intervention programs that aim to increase optimal aging. If individuals remain in denial or use avoidance behavior for too long, then health professionals might assist in moving clients out of denial and into active behavioral or cognitive coping. To the extent that cognitive coping can be beneficial, older adults with chronic disease might learn strategies that help them think through and accept unchangeable conditions.[6] As some researchers have recently pointed out, the time may have come to close the gap between coping research and clinical interventions (Coyne & Racioppo, 2000).

Because chronic diseases have become more prevalent, individuals, families, and society must prepare for effective ways to cope with chronic diseases, especially for older adults. The chapters by Poon et al., Basford et al., and Penrod et al. have given us a good start on the literature of coping with chronic disease in older adults, as well as qualitative and quantitative data that help to us understand what needs to be

---

[6]William Rakowski suggested that the objective of coping intervention might be to fit the resources of the intervention to the resources that a person has available in order to meet the demands of a specific context.

considered when building models of coping and implementing effective programs of adaptation. How can older persons age successfully when they have chronic disease? Perhaps successful aging should not be defined by the absence of disease but rather by the way people cope with the disease. As we learn more about multiple chronic conditions, we should continue to promote the highest quality of life for those whose health is, and may remain, compromised.

Chapter 11

Metanarratives Surrounding Successful Aging: The Medium Is the Message

Ann L. Whall and Frank D. Hicks

M arshall McLuhan reportedly held that, "the medium is the message." Accordingly, viewed as a whole, this book may be seen as the medium (or substantive content) that embodies an important message. The message is that many, if not most, differences in scientific inquiry are rooted in disparity among the philosophy of science positions held by those within a discourse. These differences are especially notable in cross-disciplinary fields such as gerontology. The chapters in this book suggest that several different philosophy of science positions undergird the differences between the past and present conceptualizations of successful aging.

This chapter presents three major philosophy of science positions and relates them to successful aging in general and to selected aspects of chapters within this book. When a narrative external to a given discussion is used to reinterpret that discussion, the process is termed a *metanarrative analysis* (Reed, 1995). The following is therefore a metanarrative analysis of the discussions of the concept of successful aging previously presented. The structure used for this analysis is similar to one previously presented by Whall and Hicks (2002).

Three Philosophy of Science Positions

Some 20 years ago, McKee (1982) found that various philosophy of science positions are inherent within theories of aging; he also suggested that these positions were not well recognized, which led to many differences of opinion in the study of aging. However, McKee indicated that research alone would not resolve such problems (pp. 299–301), and that once research has begun, a philosophic position has already been accepted. McKee's work can be interpreted to mean that philosophic discussions, such as those included in this chapter, should help clarify interdisciplinary efforts to define successful aging.

The three major positions that are used in this analysis are based on the early work of Kuhn (1970) and that of Lakatos (1977), and Laudan (1977). Kuhn's work, although initially spurned by the scientific community, is now generally well accepted and believed to encompass several valid points regarding scientific inquiry.

One of Kuhn's major points was that each scientific field gradually builds a body of assumptions regarding the best way to conduct science and that these assumptions are rooted in a preferred philosophy-of-science position. Thus, "truth criteria" evolve that are often unchallenged but greatly affect both the scientific processes and the products found acceptable by that science. According to Kuhn, such views are held for varying periods of time, and although largely unspoken and unrecognized, gradually evolve over time. These differences in inherent assumptions and beliefs result in the discussants' speaking past one another or overlooking newer and more fruitful ways to address a given area.

Positivism: A Difference in Focus

Positivism, one variation of which was logical positivism, dominated scientific thought from the mid-nineteenth to the mid-twentieth century. Both the Cartesian mind–body dichotomy and Kant's attempt to delineate the boundaries between science, morality, and art have been identified as driving forces behind the development of positivism (Bohm, 2000; Schrag, 1997). Positivists were committed to observing phenomena objectively, rather than utilizing metaphysical and seemingly less restrictive explanations in scientific discussions. Indeed, proponents of positivism eschewed topics and issues that could not be observed directly through the senses or objectively quantified (Scriven, 1969). This rejection of the metaphysical was a reaction in part to the philosophical movement of idealism, which promulgated the idea that science should answer metaphysical questions by asking "why," not just "how" (Carnap, 1995).

One of the major tenets of logical positivism is the verification principle, which means that phenomena are scientifically meaningful only if they are empirically verifiable via sense experience or by logical proof and mathematics (Phillips, 1987). Consequently, positivism became known for its tendency to reduce phenomena to their most simple or particulate level (reductionism), its insistence on operationalization and quantification, and its belief that there is a single 'truth' (Bohm & Peat, 2000). Positivism gained popularity because it was an important advance over earlier scientific methods of explaining things, which were less rooted in observable phenomena. Positivism was thus well accepted in the natural sciences and later within other scientific disciplines.

Within many disciplines today, a positivist worldview (or at least a strong tendency towards it) is still the ideal, so certain data such as individuals' subjective feelings are considered unimportant or invalid in scientific discussions. Instead, data sources such as laboratory test results are sought because they are seen as being more objective in nature (Giroux, 1981; Halfpenny, 1982; Lincoln & Guba, 1985; Forbes et al., 1999; Gortner, 1993). Yet positivism is criticized for relying too much on such particulate data with little attempt to provide a more holistic approach for studying phenomena (Bohm, 2000).

Several assumptions of positivism appear to be operant in the discussions of successful aging. For example, positivism values objective, directly observable data verified through the observer's senses, whereas discussions of successful aging of late have sought the opinions of the observed, that is, older persons. Likewise, because positivism holds that the arbiter of worthwhile data is the scientist, the subject's opinion is held as subjective and is, in a strict positivist view, the type of data to be eliminated. Because laboratory or bench data are considered prime within the positivist view, there is an emphasis on more particulate data than on the subject as a whole. A positivist exploration of successful aging therefore would not deal with the subject's own views of this process. As initially conceptualized, successful aging also may have been criticized as too abstract (or perhaps too holistic) from a positivist stance, and in some way denying the need to focus on multiple types of more particulate data. It is posited here that the concept of successful aging as originally proposed was a more holistic view of aging and thus conflicted with particulate or more positivist views predominant in science at that time.

Postmodernism: The Focus Extended

Postmodernism made its appearance within scientific discussions some-time around the beginning of the 20th century, although it was not generally recognized or seen as influential until the latter half of the century. As a movement, postmodernism is not easily defined because there is no singularly identified school of thought from which it emerged (Cheek, 2000). Indeed, if postmodernism has a unifying theme at all, it is diversity. Postmodernist critiques of positivism reject-ed the universal totality claims regarding rationality, the utility of grand theories, and the emphasis on a singular scientific truth (Abbey, 2000; Cheek, 2000; Schrag, 1997). Postmodern thinking is therefore a reac-tion to the more restrictive approach of positivism, such as the "con-text stripping" perspective. Under the influence of postmodernism, qualitative data (or what positivists might term *subjective data,* such as the culture and beliefs of subjects) became acceptable as scientific data.

Even though the opinions of older adult subjects are now sought with regard to what successful aging means, culture as a specific aspect of this phenomenon has yet to be well identified and addressed. The view presented in this chapter is that the initial description of success-ful aging was more consistent with the newer and broader focus of science and thus posed a problem for those with more restrictive views of science. More latitude within the broader view had led to the inclu-sion of subjects' beliefs and opinions regarding successful aging.

As with positivism, however, the new found freedom of postmodern-ism was not without criticism. The postmodern view was and is criti-cized as relativistic, irrational, nihilistic, and deconstructionist in method (Best & Kellner, 1991; Reed, 1995). There was and is a ten-dency for postmodernists to overanalyze and deconstruct, and yet pro-vide few alternatives for reconstruction. This tendency has led some to describe the deconstructionist activities of postmodernism as nihilistic or as producing a seemingly "bottomless swamp" of inadequate knowl-edge (Rolfe, 1999).

It is our view that in order to understand this newer concept of successful aging better, researchers have engaged in some overanaly-sis, which led to deconstructionist outcomes. Walker and Avant (1995) assert that early attempts to expand knowledge (as with the concept of successful aging) need to be considered in a permissive manner so as not to preempt the development of newer, more innovative theory; such latitude would suspend harsher criticism until the theory is more fully developed. To some extent, it appears that Walker and Avant's understanding has only recently held with regard to successful aging.

Neomodernism: A Possible Accommodation

The relative influence and seeming shift within the scientific paradigm or worldview from positivism to postmodernism, and more recently to neomodernism, has been a topic of discussion for several years. Kuhn (1970) observed that the development of science was not a linear process that moved smoothly from one discovery to another, nor was scientific knowledge necessarily cumulative. Scientists in Kuhn's view worked under long-held assumptions, using tried and true theories and methods—a paradigm under which "normal science" occurred. At some point, however, these assumptions, theories, and methods were believed to no longer provide sufficient explanatory or predictive power in the face of new and often serendipitous findings.

Ultimately, Kuhn (1970) believed that the new paradigm or worldview would supplant the former in a radically different way, the switch being so drastic that the new view (as well its theories and methods) would be incommensurable with the old. This thesis, however, was a problematic aspect of Kuhn's view (Phillips, 1987) because it suggested that a smooth transition from prior knowledge to newer understanding could not occur.

In terms of successful aging, if the incommensurability principle had held, more particulate data concerning successful aging (such as inclusion of physiologic findings) would have been rejected as irrelevant. This rejection has not occurred. An overview of successful aging discussions suggests that earlier knowledge is still drawn upon and is seen as foundational to current understandings of successful aging.

Stimulated by Kuhn's historicist approach, neomodernist philosophers like Laudan and Lakatos began to focus on science as a process, rather than as just a product. Laudan (1977), for example, saw science as progressing along research traditions, with a collection of assumptions, tools, methods, and axioms guiding it. Within these traditions resided many theories that could change remarkably over time, but commonalties remained that were sometimes grounded in the former research traditions. Thus, Laudan rejected the notion of incommensurability and asserted that research traditions do overlap. The hallmark of scientific progress in Laudan's view would be the transformation of anomalous and unsolved problems into solutions.

Similarly, Lakatos (1977) believed that science existed to solve the most perplexing problems, and therefore science (including theoretical and methodological aspects) must reflect sufficient diversity that is oriented toward problem solving. Theories and methods are seen as helpful if they are consistent with a specific scientific goal and need not necessarily conform to the overall paradigm accepted within a given area. Indeed, given the complexity of aging, including the notion of successful aging, it seems that an approach embracing diversity of theory and method would more likely result in solutions to problems applicable across a variety of situations.

Thus for Laudan and Lakatos, discussions of theory and method are, in the end, irrelevant. What matters is the degree to which research traditions and programs solve scientifically perplexing and socially important questions, such as the nature of successful aging. The implications of these neomodernist views for successful aging research are clear; that is, addressing successful aging with a multiplicity of theories and methods is not only desirable but will likely lead to better and clearer ways of understanding aging.

In a neomodernist world, a diversity of viewpoints is not considered negative but a normal state of science, which can lead to multiple and more adequate "ways of knowing." Such an expansion of scientific knowledge may incorporate aesthetic, ethical, and personal (experiential knowledge) as well as empirical data (Carper, 1978). Given the neomodernist trend, which seeks to understand the wholeness of a phenomenon (Bohm, 2000), a more diverse approach to the scientific study of successful aging should result in its clearer understanding.

Discussions of Successful Aging Within This Book

This book presents a diversity of opinion about successful aging that Laudan and Lakatos would view as characteristic of the neomodern era. One would expect, therefore, that multiple methods such as subject opinion surveys as well as reanalysis of large data sets would be represented. This is indeed the case in this text. Recognizing the importance of this variety, we have not categorized chapters as presenting any one philosophy of science position. It is also the case that in the current era, no one philosophy of science is necessarily considered superior to another. Rather, the question is, Superior for what purpose? Analysis of these positions, however, should provide alternatives for better understanding the development of the diverse theory underlying the study of successful aging.

In light of this historical discourse on successful aging, Strawbridge and Wallhagen (chapter 1) asked older persons to rate themselves on successful aging, surveying a sample from the Alameda County Study. Because postmodernism sought to avoid context stripping, it can be said that the authors' approach is characteristic of the broadened perspective of postmodernism. In their study, Strawbridge and Wallhagen suggest that persons must be considered within their contextual environment and consulted in terms of their own beliefs.

Strawbridge and Wallhagen also point out that the concept of successful aging has changed and broadened over the years. They explain that there are several ways that successful aging has been conceptualized, for example, as a person's having no decline in physiologic functioning, as not demonstrating decrements due to illness, and other criteria. Strawbridge and Wallhagen note that as definitions of successful aging have broadened, they have included such aspects as maintenance of physical and mental functioning and being actively engaged with life. Inclusion of these aspects in the definition of successful aging presents a much broader view.

Indeed, the broadening conceptualization of successful aging suggests a trend toward a postmodern perspective, and perhaps a movement toward the more diverse perspective of neomodernism as well. Self-evaluation of a subject's coping efforts are, for example, arguably based on aesthetic and ethical preferences as well as on cultural mores. Thus, someone with a genetic predisposition for dementia might mitigate this genetic heritage through the use of aesthetic and physiologic means, based on their ethical reasoning and personal experience.

Although the neomodernist perspective is not as yet fully explicated, descriptions suggest the inclusion of a variety of ways of knowing for concepts such as successful aging. Such a perspective on successful aging is consistent with Strawbridge and Wallhagen's views (citing Baltes & Baltes, 1990b) as "doing the best one can with what one has."

In the same regard, Rakowski, Clark, Miller, and Berg (chapter 2) discuss plasticity by addressing the psychological processes of aging, adding depth to the discussions of successful aging and extending the discussions beyond a deficit model. One of their points is that persons with multiple illnesses and functional impairments are not necessarily or automatically aging "unsuccessfully." Within this view, perhaps empirical data alone would not adequately have defined successful aging.

Rakowski et al. further address successful aging in terms of reciprocity among older adults in assisted living settings. The term reciprocity indicates a fully interactive relationship between a person and his or her environment as well as between the observed and the observer, a rather postmodern norm. Within this perspective the observer no longer judges the situation as either successful or unsuccessful since an open system (such as a person) is not adequately described in dichotomous terms alone. Far from the controlled experiment favored by positivism, Rakowski et al. describe observations using a more open perspective, which provides more alternatives with which to approach successful aging.

Poon et al. (chapter 7) ask, "What is comorbidity?" and "What do we know about coping with comorbidity among older adults?" From an arguably postmodern position, they examined successful aging in terms of how older adults cope with comorbidity; they searched 12 data bases and found two distinct paradigms with regard to coping, that is, biologic and epidemiologic. With the inclusion of epidemiology, there is an extension beyond person to community, a broadened perspective requiring synthesis of knowledge. Likewise Crimmins et al. (chapter 4) discuss the term "health expectancy" that also allows for the consideration of proactive health practices regardless of existing conditions, a seeming extension of a postmodern position. As a whole, therefore, the chapters of this text vary in philosophy-of-science positions, but generally they present a more broadened view of successful aging and a variety of newer ways by which to understand and explore this phenomenon.

Conclusions

McKee points out that philosophy of science positions, although largely unrecognized, underlie multiple issues in aging theory and research. The conceptualization of successful aging has broadened over time and is reflective of different aspects of philosophy of science positions, although this influence is still largely unrecognized. Discussion of differing views associated with these positions, may help avoid some of the past problems identified in discussions of successful aging, and hopefully support multiple ways in which to further develop the concept.

References

Abbey, R. (2000). Charles Taylor: Philosophy now. In J. Shand (Series Ed.), *Philosophy now*. Princeton, NJ: Princeton & Oxford Press.

Abeles, R. P., Gift, H. G., & Ory, M. G. (Eds.). (1994). *Aging and quality of life*. New York: Springer.

Adams, P. F., & Marrano, M. A. (1995). Current estimates from the National Health Interview Survey, 1994. *Vital Health Statistics, 10*, (193). Hyattsville, MD: National Center for Health Statistics.

Affleck, G., & Tennen, H. (1992). Neuroticism and the pain-mood relation in rheumatoid arthritis: Insights from a prospective daily study. *Journal of Consulting and Clinical Psychology, 60*, 119–126.

Affleck, G., Urrows, S., Tennen, H., & Higgins, P. (1992). Daily coping with pain from rheumatoid arthritis: Patterns and correlates. *Pain, 51*, 221–229.

Agrawal, A., & Pandey, A. (1998). Coping with chronic disease: Role of psychosocial variables. *Psychological Studies, 43*(1–2), 58–64.

Ai, A. L., Peterson, C., & Boiling, S. F. (1997). Psychological recovery from coronary artery bypass graft surgery: The use of complementary therapies. *Journal of Alternative and Complementary Medicine, 3*, 343–353.

Albert, M. S., Jones, K., Savage, C. R., Berkman, L., Seeman, T., Blazer, D., et al. (1995). Predictors of cognitive change in older persons: The MacArthur Studies of Successful Aging. *Psychology and Aging, 10*, 578–589.

Aldwin, C. M., Sutton, K. J., Chiara, G., & Spiro, A. (1996). Age differences in stress, coping, and appraisal: Findings from the Normative Aging Study. *Journals of Gerontology, Series B: Psychological Sciences and Social Sciences, 51B*, 179–188.

Alexopoulos, G. S., Vrontou, C., Kakuma, T., Meyers, B. S., Young, R. C., Klausner, L. E., & Clarkin, J. (1996). Disability in geriatric depression. *American Journal of Psychiatry, 153*, 877–885.

American Association of Home and Services for the Aging. (1999). What is assisted living? [on-line]. Available: www.aahsa.org

American Psychiatric Association. (1994). *Diagnostic and statistical manual of mental disorders* (4th ed.). Washington, DC: Author.

Angel, R. J., & Angel, J. L. (1995). Mental and physical comorbidity among the elderly: The role of culture and social class. In D. K. Padgett (Ed.), *Handbook on ethnicity, aging, and mental health* (pp. 47–70). Westport, CT: Greenwood.

Antonucci, T. C. (1985). Personal characteristics, social support and social behavior. In B. E. Shanas (Ed.), *Aging and the social sciences*. New York: Van Nostrand Reinhold.

Arling, G. (1987). Strain, social support, and distress in old age. *Journal of Gerontology, 42*(1), 107–113.

Armor, D. J., Polich, M., & Stambul, H. B. (1975). *Alcoholism and treatment.* New York: Wiley.

Arnold, M. S., Butler, P. M., Anderson, R. M., Funnell, M. M., & Feste, C. (1995). Guidelines for facilitating a patient empowerment program. *Diabetes Educator, 21,* 308–312.

Assisted Living Federation of America. (2002). ALFA Online. What is assisted living? [on-line]. www.alfa.org

Baker, C., & Stern, P. N. (1993). Finding meaning in chronic illness as the key to self-care. *Canadian Journal of Nursing Research, 25,* 23–36.

Baltes, M. M. (1994). Aging well and institutional living: A paradox? In R. P. Abeles, H. C. Gift, & M. G. Ory (Eds.), *Aging and quality of life* (pp. 185–201). New York: Springer.

Baltes, P. B. (1997). On the incomplete architecture of human ontogeny: Selection, optimization, and compensation as foundation of developmental theory. *American Psychologist,* 366–380.

Baltes, P. B., & Baltes, M. M. (1990a). Psychological perspectives on successful aging: The model of selective optimization with compensation. In P. B. Baltes & M. M. Baltes (Eds.), *Successful aging: Perspectives from the behavioral sciences* (pp. 1–34). New York: Cambridge University Press.

Baltes, P. B., & Baltes, M. M. (1990b). *Successful aging: Perspectives from the behavioral sciences.* Cambridge, UK: Cambridge University Press.

Baltes, M. M., & Carstensen, L. L. (1996). The process of successful aging. *Aging and Society, 16,* 397–422.

Barkwell, D. P. (1991). Ascribed meaning: A critical factor in coping and pain attenuation in patients with cancer-related pain. *Journal of Palliative Care, 7*(3), 5–14.

Bartmann, J. A., & Roberto, K. A. (1996). Coping strategies of middle-aged and older women who have undergone a mastectomy. *Journal of Applied Gerontology, 15,* 376–386.

Basford, L., Nyatanga, L., & Dann, K. (2001). *Empowerment in the field of mental health care.* Derby, UK: University of Derby.

Bazargan, M. (1996). Self-reported sleep disturbance among African-American elderly: The effects of depression, health status, exercise, and social support. *International Journal of Aging and Human Development, 42*(2), 143–160.

Beehr, T. A., & McGrath, J. E. (1996). The methodology of research on coping: Conceptual, strategic, and operational-level issues. In M. Zeidner & N. S. Endler (Eds.), *Handbook of coping* (pp. 65–82). New York: Wiley.

Belgrave, F. Z., & Lewis, D. M. (1994). The role of social support in compliance and other health behaviors for African Americans with chronic illnesses. *Journal of Health Social Policy, 5,* 55–68.

Benfante, R., Reed., D., & Brody, J. (1985). Biological and social predictors of health in an aging cohort. *Journal of Chronic Disease, 38,* 385–395.

Bennahum, D. A., Forman, W. B., Vellas, B., & Albarede, J. L. (1997). Life expectancy, comorbidity, and quality of life: A framework of reference for medical decisions. *Clinics in Geriatric Medicine, 13,* 33–53.

Bennett, P. E., Weinman, J. D., & Spurgeon, P. E. (1990). *Current developments in health psychology.* London: Harwood.

Berckman, K. L., & Austin, J. K. (1993). Causal attribution, perceived control, and adjustment in patients with lung cancer. *Oncology Nursing Forum, 20*(1), 23–30.

Bergstrom, M. J., & Holmes, M .E. (2000). Lay theories of successful aging after the death of a spouse: A network text analysis of bereavement advice. *Health Communication, 12,* 377–406.

Berkman, L. F., & Breslow, L. (1983). *Health and ways of living: The Alameda County Study.* New York: Oxford University Press.

Berkman, L. F., Leo-Summers, L., & Horwitz, R. I. (1992). Emotional support and survival after myocardial infarction: A prospective, population-based study of the elderly. *Annals of Internal Medicine, 117,* 1003–1009.

Berkman, L. F., Seeman, T. E., Albert, M., Blazer, D., Kahn, R., Mohs, R., Finch, C., Schneider, E., et al. (1993). High, usual and impaired functioning in community-dwelling older men and women: Findings from the MacArthur Foundation Research Network on Successful Aging. *Journal of Clinical Epidemiology, 46,* 1129–40.

Bergstrom, M. J., & Holmes, M. E. (2000). Lay theories of successful aging after the death of a spouse: A network text analysis of bereavement advice. *Health Communication, 12,* 377–406.

Berman, A., & Studenski, S. (1998). Musculoskeletal rehabilitation. *Clinics in Geriatric Medicine, 14,* 641–659.

Best, S., & Kellner, D. (1991). *Postmodern theory: Critical interrogations.* New York: Guilford.

Blair, S. N., Kohl, H. W., III, Barlow, C. E., Pfaffenbarger, R. S., Jr., Gibbons, L. W., & Macera, C. A. (1995). Changes in physical fitness and all-cause mortality. *Journal of the American Medical Association, 273,* 1093–1098.

Blake, R. L., Jr., Vandiver, T. A., Braun, S., Bertuso, D. D., & Straub, V. (1990). A randomized controlled evaluation of a psychosocial intervention in adults with chronic lung disease. *Family Medicine, 22,* 365–370.

Bohm, D. (2000). *Wholeness and the implicate order.* New York: Routledge.

Bohm, D., & Peat, F. D. (2000). *Science, order, and creativity* (2nd ed.). New York: Routledge.

Bombardier, C. H., D'Amico, C., & Jordan, J. S. (1990). The relationship of appraisal and coping to chronic illness adjustment. *Behaviour Research and Therapy, 28,* 297–304.

Bradburn, N. M. (1969). *This structure of psychological well-being.* Chicago: Aldine.

Brody, E., & Kleban, M. (1983). Day-to-day mental and physical health symptoms of older people: A report on health logs. *Gerontologist, 23,* 75–85.

Broe, G. A., Jorm, A. F., Creasey, H., Grayson, D., Edeibrock, D., Waite, L. M., Bennett, H., Cullen, J. S., & Casey, B. (1998). Impact of chronic systemic and neurological disorders on disability, depression and life satisfaction. *International Journal of Geriatric Psychiatry, 10,* 667–673.

Brown, G. K., & Nicassio, P. M. (1987). Development of a questionnaire for the assessment of active and passive coping strategies in chronic pain patients. *Pain, 31,* 53–64.

Brown, G. K., Wallston, K.A., & Nicassio, P. M. (1989). Social support and depression in rheumatoid arthritis: A one-year prospective study. *Journal of Applied Social Psychology, 19,* 1164–1181.

Burke, M., & Flaherty, M. J. (1993). Coping strategies and health status of elderly arthritic women. *Journal of Advanced Nursing, 18,* 7–13.

Burnette, D., & Mui, A. C. (1994). Determinants of self-reported depressive symptoms by frail elderly persons living alone. *Journal of Gerontological Social Work, 22,*(1–2) 3–19.

Bush, T. L., Miller, S. R., Golden, A. L., & Hale, W. E. (1989). Self-report and medical record report agreement of selected medical conditions in the elderly. *American Journal of Public Health, 79,* 1554–1556.

Butler, R. N. (1974). Successful aging. *Mental Health, 58,* 6–12.

Butler, R. N., Davis, R., Lewis, C. B., Nelson, M. E., & Strauss, E. (1998). Physical fitness: Benefits of exercise for the older patient. Part 2 of a roundtable discussion. *Geriatrics, 53,* 46–52.

Butler, R. N., & Gleason, H. P. (Eds.). (1985). *Productive aging: Enhancing vitality in later life.* New York: Springer.

Cantril, H. (1965). *The pattern of human concerns.* New Brunswick, NJ: Rutgers University Press.

Carnap, R. (1995). *An introduction to the philosophy of science.* New York: Dover.

Carper, B. (1978). Fundamental patterns of knowing in nursing. *Advances in Nursing Science, 1,* 13–23.

Carruth, A. K., & Boss, B. J. (1990). More than they bargained for: Adverse drug effects. *Journal of Gerontological Nursing, 16,* 27–31.

Charlson, M. E., Pompei, P., Ales, K. L., & MacKenzie, C. R. (1987). A new method of classifying prognostic comorbidity in longitudinal studies: Development and validation. *Journal of Chronic Health Conditions, 40,* 373–383.

Cheek, J. (2000). *Postmodern and poststructural approaches to nursing research.* Thousand Oaks, CA: Sage.

Clark, F., Carison, M., Zemke, R., Gelya, F., Patterson, K., Ennevor, B. L., et al. (1996). Life domains and adaptive strategies of a group of low-income, well older adults. *American Journal of Occupational Therapy, 50*(2), 99–108.

Colantonio, A., Kasi, S. V., Ostfeld, A. M., & Berkman, L. F. (1993). Psychosocial predictors of stroke outcomes in an elderly population. *Journal of Gerontology, 48,* S261–S268.

Cook, N. R., Evans, D. A., Scherr, P. A., Speizer, F. E., Taylor, J. O., & Hennekens, C. H. (1991). Peak expiratory flow rate and 5-year mortality in an elderly poopulation. *American Journal of Epidemiology, 33,* 784–794.

Cook, W. W., & Medley, D. M. (1954). Proposed hostility and pharisaic-virtue scales for the MMPI. *Journal of Applied Psychology, 38,* 414–418.

Coroni-Huntley, J. C., Brock, D. B., Ostfeld, A. M., Taylor, J. O., & Wallace, R. B. (Eds.). (1986). *Established populations for epidemiologic studies of the elderly* NIH Publication No. 86–2443, pp. Washington, DC: National Institutes of Aging.

Coyne, J. C., & Bolger, N. (1990). Doing without social support as an explanatory concept. *Journal of Social and Clinical Psychology, 9*(1), 148–158.

Coyne, J. C., & DeLongis, A. (1986). Going beyond social support: The role of social relationships in adaptation. *Journal of Consulting and Clinical Psychology, 54,* 454–460.

Coyne, J. C., & Racioppo, M. W. (2000). Never the twain shall meet? Closing the gap between coping research and clinical intervention research. *American Psychologist, 5,* 655–664.

Craig, H. M., & Edwards, J. E. (1983). Adaptation in chronic illness: An eclectic model for nurses. *Journal of Advanced Nursing, 8,* 397–404.

Cramer, P. (2000). Defense mechanisms in psychology today: Further process for adaptation. *American Psychologist, 55,* 637–646.

Crimmins, E., Saito, Y., & Ingegneri, D. (1989). Changes in life expectancy and disability-free life expectancy in the United Status. *Population and Development Review, 15,* 235–267.

Crimmins, E., Saito, Y., & Ingegneri, D. (1997). Trends in disability-free life expectancy in the United States, 1970–1990. *Population and Development Review, 23,* 555–572.

Cumming, E., & Henry, W. E. (1961). *Growing old.* New York: Basic Books.

Dargent-Molina, P., Hays, M., & Breart, G. (1996). Sensory impairments and physical disability in aged women living at home. *International Journal of Epidemiology, 25,* 621–629.

Davidson, G. C., Williams, M. E., Nezami, E., Bice, T. L., & DeQuattro, V. L. (1991). Relaxation, reduction in angry articulated thoughts, and improvements in borderline hypertension and heart rate. *Journal of Behavioral Medicine, 14,* 453–468.

Degazon, C. E. (1995). Coping, diabetes, and the older African American. *Nursing Outlook, 43,* 254–259.

De Klerk, M. M. Y., Huijsman, R., & McDonnell, J. (1997). The use of technical aids by elderly persons in the Netherlands: An application of the Andersen and Newman Model. *Gerontologist, 37,* 365–373.

DeMaria, L., & Cohen, H. J. (1987). Characteristics of lung cancer in elderly patients. *Journal of Gerontology, 42,* 185–190.

Department of Health. (1989). Caring for people-community care in the next decade and beyond. Cm. 849, London: HMSO.

de Ridder, D., Depla, M., Severens, P., & Malsch, M. (1997). Beliefs on coping with illness: A consumer's perspective. *Social Science and Medicine, 44,* 553–559.

de Ridder, D. T. D., & Schreurs, K. M. G. (1994). Coping en sociale steun van chronisch zieken [Coping and social support in patients with chronic diseases]. Report for the Dutch Commission for Chronic Diseases. Utrecht, The Netherlands: Section of Clinical and Health Psychology.

Derogatis, L. R., Lipman, R. S., Rickels, K., Uhlenhuth, E. H., & Covi, L. (1974). The Hopkins Symptom Checklist (HSCL): A self-report symptom inventory. *Behavioral Science, 19,* 1–15.

Diehl, M. (1998). Everyday competence in later life: Current status and future directions. *Gerontologist, 38,* 422–433.

Do Rozario, L. (1997). Spirituality in the lives of people with disability and chronic illness: A creative paradigm of wholeness and reconstitution, disability and rehabilitation. *International Multidisciplinary Journal, 19,* 427–434.

Dowd, J. J. (1975). Aging as exchange: A preface to theory. *Journal of Gerontology, 30,* 584–594.

Dowd, J. J. (1980). Exchange rates and old people. *Journal of Gerontology, 35,* 596–602.

Dowdy, S. W., Dwyer, K. A., Smith, C. A., & Wallston, K. A. (1996). Gender and psychological well-being of persons with rheumatoid arthritis. *Arthritis Care and Research, 9,* 449–456.

DowneWamboldt, B. L., & Melanson, P. M. (1995). Emotions, coping, and psychological well-being in elderly people with arthritis. *Western Journal of Nursing Research, 17,* 250–265.

Dowzer, C., Basford, L., Booth, A., & Poon, L. W. (1999). *Living with multiple health conditions: A systematic search and literature review.* Unpublished manuscript, University of Sheffield, England, and University of Georgia, Athens.

Dunkle, R. (1985). Comparing the depression of elders in two types of caregiving arrangements. *Family Relations, 34,* 235–240.

Eakes, G. G. (1993). Chronic sorrow: A response to living with cancer. *Oncology Nursing Forum, 20,* 1327–1334.

Eizenman, D. R., Nesselroade, J. R., Featherman, D. L., & Rowe, J. W. (1997). Intra-individual variability in perceived control in an older sample: The MacArthur Studies of Successful Aging. *Psychology and Aging, 12,* 489–502.

Endler, N. S., Courbasson, C. M. A., & Fillion, L. (1998). Coping with cancer: The evidence for the temporal stability of the French-Canadian version of Coping with Health Injuries and Problems (CHIP). *Personality and Individual Differences, 25,* 711–717.

Erdal, K. J., & Zautra, A. J. (1995). Psychological impact of illness downturns: A comparison of new and chronic conditions. *Psychology and Aging, 10,* 570–577.

Erickson, H., & Swain, M. A. (1990). Mobilizing self-care resources: A nursing intervention for hypertension. *Issues in Mental Health Nursing, 11,* 217–235.

Erickson, P., Wilson, R., & Shannon, I. (1995). *Years of healthy life: Healthy People 2000 Statistical Notes, No 7.* Hyattsville, MD: National Center for Health Statistics.

Evans, M. E., Copeland, J. R., & Dewey, M. E. (1991). Depression in the elderly in the community: Effect of physical illness and selected social factors. *International Journal of Geriatric Psychiatry, 6,* 787–795.

Evers, A. W. M., Kraaimaat, F. W., Geenen, R., & Bijlsma, J. W. J. (1998). Psychosocial predictors of functional change in recently diagnosed rheumatoid arthritis patients. *Behavior Research and Therapy, 36,* 179–193.

Everson, S. A., Kauhanen, J., Kaplan, G. A., Goldberg, D. E., Julkunen, J., Tuomilehto, J., et al. (1997). Hostility and increased risk of mortality and acute myocardial infarction: The mediating role of behavioral risk factors. *American Journal of Epidemiology, 146,* 142–152.

Falvo, D. R. (1991). *Medical and psychosocial aspects of chronic illness and disability.* Gaithersburg, MD: Aspen.

Featherman, D. L., Smith, J., & Peterson, J. G. (1990). Successful aging in a post-retired society. In P. B. Baltes & M. M. Baltes (Eds.), *Successful aging: Perspectives from the behavioral sciences* (pp. 50–93). New York: Cambridge University Press.

Feifel, H., Strack, S., & Nagy, V. T. (1987a). Coping strategies and associated features of medically ill patients. *Psychosomatic Medicine, 49,* 616–625.

Feifel, H., Strack, S., & Nagy, V. T. (1987b). Degree of life-threat and differential use of coping modes. *Journal of Psychosomatic Research, 31,* 91–99.

Feinstein, A. R. (1970). The pre-therapeutic classification of comorbidity in chronic disease. *Journal of Chronic Health Conditions, 23,* 455–457.

Felton, B. J. (1990). Coping and social support in older people's experiences of chronic illness. In M. Stephens, A. Parris, & J. H. E. Crowther (Eds.), *Stress and coping in later-life families* (pp. 153–171). New York: Hemisphere.

Felton, B. J., & Revenson, T. A. (1987). Age differences in coping with chronic illness. *Psychology and Aging, 2,* 164–170.

Fisher, B. (1995). Successful aging, life satisfaction, and generativity in later life. *International Journal of Aging and Human Development, 41,* 239–250.

Fitzgerald, R. G., & Parkes, G. M. (1998). Blindness and loss of other sensory and cognitive functions. *British Medical Journal, 316,* 1160–1163.

Folden, S. L. (1990). On the inside looking out: Perceptions of the homebound. *Journal of Gerontological Nursing, 16,* 9–15.

Folkman, S., & Lazarus, R. S. (1980). An analysis of coping in a middle-aged community sample. *Journal of Health and Social Behavior, 21,* 219–239.

Folkman, S., & Lazarus, R. S. (1988). *Manual for the Ways of Coping Questionnaire.* Palo Alto, CA: Consulting Psychologists.

Folkman, S., Lazarus, R. S., Pimley, S., & Novacek, J. (1987). Age differences in stress and coping processes. *Psychology of Aging, 2,* 171–184.

Folkman, S., & Moskowitz, J. T. (2000). Positive affect and the other side of coping. *American Psychologist, 55,* 647–654.

Forbes, D., King, K., Kushner, K., Letourneau, N., Myrick, A., & Profetto-McGrath, J. (1999). Warrantable evidence in nursing science. *Journal of Advanced Nursing, 29,* 373–379.

Forette, B. (1999). Are common risk factors relevant in the eldest old? In J. Robine, B. Forette, C. Franceschi, & M. Allard (Eds.), *The paradoxes of longevity* (pp. 73–79). New York: Springer.

Frazer, D. W., Leicht, M. L., & Baker, M. D. (1996). Psychological manifestations of physical disease in the elderly. In L. E. Carstensen (Ed.), *The practical handbook of clinical gerontology* (pp. 217–235). Thousand Oaks, CA: Sage.

Freedland, K. E., Camey, R. M., Rich, M. W., Caracciolo, A., Krotenberg, J. A., Smith, L. J., et al. (1991). Depression in elderly patients with congestive heart failure. *Journal of Geriatric Psychiatry, 24,* 59–71.

Frenzel, M. P., McCaul, K. D., Glasgow, R. E., & Schafer, L. C. (1988). The relationship of stress and coping to regimen adherence and glycemic control of diabetes. *Journal of Social and Clinical Psychology, 6,* 77–87.

Fried, L. P., BandeenRoche, K., Kaser, J. D., & Guralnik, J. M. (1999). Association of comorbidity with disability in older women: The women's health and aging study. *Journal of Clinical Epidemiology, 52,* 27–37.

Fried, L. P., & Guralnik, J. M. (1997). Disability in older adults: Evidence regarding significance, etiology, and risk. *Journal of the American Geriatrics Society, 45,* 92–100.

Fries, J. F. (1983). The compression of morbidity. *Milbank Memorial Fund Quarterly, 61,* 130–136.

Fries, J. F., & Crapo, L. F. (1981). *Vitality and aging: Implications of the rectangular curve.* San Francisco: Freeman.

Fry, P. S., & Wong, T. P. (1991). Pain management training in the elderly: Matching interventions with subjects' coping styles. *Stress Medicine, 7,* 93–98.

Gambassi, G., Lapane, K., Sgadari, A., Landi, F., Carbonin, P., Hume, A., et al. (1998). Prevalence, clinical correlates, and treatment of hypertension in elderly nursing home residents: SAGE (Systematic Assessment of Geriatric drug use via Epidemiology) study group. *Archives of International Medicine, 158,* 2377–2385.

Gard, D., Harris, J., Edwards, P. W., & McCormack, G. (1988). Sensitizing effects of pre-treatment measures on cancer chemotherapy nausea and vomiting. *Journal of Consulting and Clinical Psychology, 56,* 30–84.

Garfein, A. J., & Herzog, A. R. (1995). Robust aging among the young-old, old-old, and oldest-old. *Journal of Gerontology: Social Sciences, 50B,* 577–587.

Gentry, W. D., Foster, S., & Haney, T. (1972). Denial as a determinant of anxiety and perceived health status in the coronary care unit. *Psychosomatic Medicine, 34,* 39–44.

Giroux, H. (1981). *Ideology, culture, and the process of schooling.* Philadelphia: Temple University Press.

Glaser, B. G., & Strauss, A. L. (1967). *The discovery of grounded theory.* Chicago: Aldine.

Glasgow, R. E., Ruggiero, L., Eakin., E. G., Dryfoos, J., & Chobanian, L. (1997). Quality of life and associated characteristics in a large national sample of adults with diabetes. *Diabetes Care, 20,* 562–567.

Gortner, S. R. (1993). Nursing's syntax revisited: Toward a science philosophy. *International Journal of Nursing Studies, 30,* 447–488.

Grady, C. L., Maisog, J. M., Horwitz, B., & Ungerleider, L. G. (1994). Age-related changes in cortical blood flow activation during visual processing of faces and location. *Journal of Neuroscience, 14,* 1450–1462.

Greenfield, S., Apolone, G., McNeil, B. J., & Cleary, P. D. (1993). The importance of co-existent disease in the occurrence of postoperative complications and one-year recovery in patients undergoing total hip replacement. *Medical Care, 31,* 141–154.

Greenglass, E. R., & Julkunen. (1989). Construct validity and sex differences in Cook-Medley hostility. *Personality and Individual Differences, 10,* 209–218.

Guralnik, J., & Kaplan, G. K. (1989). Predictors of healthy aging: Prospective evidence from the Alameda County Study. *American Journal of Public Health, 79,* 703–708.Guralnik, J. M. (1996). Assessing the impact of comorbidity in the older population. *Annals of Epidemiology, 6,* 376–380.

Guralnik, J. M., LaCroix, A. Z., Abbott, R. D., Berkman, L. F., Satterfield, S., Evans, D., et al. (1993). Maintaining mobility in late life: Demographic characteristics and chronic conditions. *American Journal of Epidemiology, 137,* 845–857.

Guralnik, J. M., & Schneider, E. L. (1987). The compression of morbidity: A dream which may come true, someday. *Gerontologica Perspecta, 1,* 8–14.

Guse, L. W., & Masesar, M. A. (1999). Quality of life and successful aging in long-term care: Perceptions of residents. *Issues in Mental Health Nursing, 20,* 527–539.

Hageman, W. J. J. M., & Arrindell, W. A. (1993). A further refinement of the reliable change (RC) index by improving the pre-post difference score: Introducing RC_{ID}. *Behavior Research and Therapy, 3,* 693–700.

Hageman, W. J. J. M., & Arrindell, W. A. (1999). Establishing clinically significant change: Increment of precision and the distinction between individual and group level of analysis. *Behavior Research and Therapy, 37,* 1169–1193.

Hahn, W. K., Brooks, J. A., & Hartsough, D. M. (1993). Self-disclosure and coping styles in men with cardiovascular reactivity. *Research in Nursing and Health, 16,* 275–282.

Hakim, A. A., Petrovitch, H., Burchfiel, C. M., Ross, W. G., Rodriguez, B. L., White, L. R., Hampson, S. E., Glasglow, R. E., & Zeiss, A. M. (1998). Personal models of osteoarthritis and their relation to self-management activities and quality of life. *Journal of Behavioral Medicine, 17,* 143–158.

Hakim, A. A., Petrovitch, H., Burchfiel, C. M., Ross, W. G., Rodriguez, B. L., White, L. R., Katsuhiko, Y., Curb, D., & Abbott, R. D. (1998). Effects of walking on mortality among nonsmoking retired men. *New England Journal of Medicine, 338,* 94–99.

Halfpenny, P. (1982). *Positivism and sociology.* London: Allen & Unwin.

Hallberg, L. R., & Carisson. S. G. (1991). A qualitative study of strategies for managing a hearing impairment. *British Journal of Audiology, 25,* 201–211.

Halstead, M. T., & Femsler, I. I. (1994). Coping strategies of long-term cancer survivors. *Cancer Nursing, 17* (2), 94–100.

Hampson, S. E., Glasgow, R. E., & Zeiss, A. M. (1994). Personal models of osteoarthritis and their relation to self-management activities and quality of life. *Journal of Behavioral Medicine, 17,* 143–158.

Hart, R. P., & Kwentus, J. A. (1987). Psychomotor slowing and subcortical type dysfunction in depression. *Journal of Neurology, Neurosurgery, and Psychiatry, 50,* 1263–1266.

Hasitavej, M. L. (1995). The impact of psychotherapy and self-healing techniques when coping with chronic illness: A case study. *Home Healthcare Nurse, 13,* 40–43.

Havighurst, R.J. (1963). Successful aging. In R. H. Williams, C. Tibbits, & W. Donahue (Eds.), *Processes of aging* (Vol. 1, pp. 299–320). New York: Atherton.

Hazzard, W. R. (1995). Weight control and exercise: Cardinal features of successful preventive gerontology [Editorial]. *Journal of the America Medical Association, 274,* 1964–1965.

Heidrich, S. M. (1996). Mechanisms related to psychological well-being in older women with chronic illnesses: Age and disease comparisons. *Research in Nursing and Health, 19,* 225–235.

Heidrich, S. M., & Ryff, C. D. (1992). How elderly women cope: Concerns and strategies. *Public Health Nursing, 9,* 200–208.

Herbert, R., & Gregor, F. (1997). Quality of life and coping strategies of clients with COPD. *Rehabilitation Nursing, 22,* 182–187.

Herzog, A. R., & Morgan, J. N. (1992). Age and gender differences in the value of productive activities: Four different approaches. *Research on Aging, 14,* 169–198.

Hickey, T., Wolf, F. M., Robins, L. S., Wagner, M. B., & Harik, W. (1995). Physical activity training for functional mobility in older persons. *Journal of Applied Gerontology, 14,* 357–371.

Hodgson, C. (1998). Prevalence and disabilities of community-living seniors who report the effects of stroke. *Canadian Medical Association, 6*(Suppl.), S9–S14.

Hoffman, C., Rice, D., & Sung, H. Y. (1996). Persons with chronic conditions: Their prevalence and costs. *Journal of the American Medical Association, 276,* 1473–1479.

Holahan, C. J., Moos, R. H., Holahan, C. K., & Brennan, P. L. (1995). Social support, coping, and depressive symptoms in a late-middle-aged sample of patients reporting cardiac illness. *Health Psychology, 14,* 152–163.

Holahan, C. J., Moos, R. H., Holahan, C. K., & Brennan, P. L. (1997). Social context, coping strategies, and depressive symptoms: An expanded model with cardiac patients. *Journal of Personality and Social Psychology, 72,* 918–928.

Holahan, C. J., Moos, R. H., & Schaefer, J. A. (1996). Coping, stress resistance, and growth: Conceptualizing adaptive functioning. In M. Zeidner & N. S. Endler (Eds.), *Handbook of coping* (pp. 24–43). New York: Wiley.

Hopman-Rock, M., Kraaimaat, F. W., Odding, E., & Bijisma, J. W. J. (1998). Coping with pain in the hip or knee in relation to physical disability in community-living elderly people. *Arthritis Care and Research, 11,* 243–252.

Horgas, A. L., Wilms, H-U., & Baltes, M. M. (1998). Daily life in very old age: Everyday activities as expression of successful living. *Gerontologist, 38,* 556–568.

Horwitz, A. V., Reinhard, S. C., & Howell-White, S. (1996). Caregiving as reciprocal exchange in families with seriously mentally ill members. *Journal of Health and Social Behavior, 37,* 149–162.

Hypertension Detection and Follow-up Program Cooperative Group (HDFP). (1978). Variability of blood pressure and results of screening in HDFP program. *Journal of Chronic Diseases, 31,* 651–667.

Ingersoll-Dayton, B., & Antonucci, T. C. (1988). Reciprocal and nonreciprocal social support: Contrasting sides of intimate relationships. *Journal of Gerontology: Social Sciences, 43,* S65–S73.

Inouye, S., Albert, M., Mohs, R.D., Sun, K., & Berkman, L. F. (1993). Cognitive performance in a high functioning community-dwelling elderly population. *Journal of Gerontology, 48,* M146–M151.

Institute of Medicine. (1990). Social isolation among older individuals: The relationship to mortality and morbidity. In R. L. Berg & J. S. Cassells (Eds.), *The second 50 years: Promoting health and preventing disability* (pp. 243–262). Washington, DC: Institute of Medicine.

Johnson, C. L., & Barber, B. M. (1999). Coping and a sense of control among the oldest old: An exploratory analysis. *Journal of Aging Studies, 7,* 67–80.

Jones, D. C., & Vaughan, K. (1990). Close friendships among senior adults. *Psychology and Aging, 5,* 451–457.

Kahana, E., & Kahana, B. (2001). Successful aging among people with HIV/AIDS. *Journal of Clinical Epidemiology, 54,* S53–S56.

Kahn, R., & Antonucci, T. (1980). Convoys over the life course: Attachment roles and social supports. In P. Baltes & O. Brim (Eds.), *Life span development and behavior* (pp. 254–283). New York: Academic Press.

Kahn, R. L. (1994). Social support: Content, causes and consequences. In R. P. Abeles, H. C. Gift, & M. G. Ory (Eds.), *Aging and the quality of life* (pp. 163–184). New York: Springer.

Kahn, R. L. (1981). *Work and health.* New York: Wiley.

Kalfoss, M. H. (1993). Coping and depression in chronically ill hospitalized elderly patients. *Nordic Journal of Psychiatry, 47,* 85–94.

Kaplan, G. A., & Strawbridge, W. J. (1994). Behavioral and social factors in healthy aging. In R. P. Abeles, H. C. Gift, & M. G. Ory (Eds.), *Aging and quality of life* (pp. 57–58). New York: Springer.

Kaplan, G. A., Strawbridge, W. J., Cohen, R. D., & Hungerford, L. H. (1996). Natural history of leisure-time physical activity and its correlates: Associations with mortality from all-causes and cardiovascular disease over 28 years. *American Journal of Epidemiology, 144,* 793–797.

Kaplan, M., & Feinstein, A. R. (1974). The importance of classifying initial comorbidity in evaluating the outcome of diabetes mellitus. *Journal of Chronic Diseases, 27,* 387–404.

Katona, C. L. E., et al. (1999). Comorbidity with depression in older people: The Islington Study. *Aging and Mental Health, 1,* 57–61.

Katz, S. C., Ford, A. B., Moskowitz, R. W., Jackson, B. A., & Jaffe, M. W. (1963). Studies of illness in the aged. The index of ADL: A standardized measure of biological and psychosocial function. *Journal of the American Medical Association, 185,* 914–919.

Keefe, F. J., Brown, G. K., Wallston, K. A., & Caldwell, D. S. (1989). Coping with rheumatoid arthritis pain: Catastrophizing as a maladaptive strategy. *Pain, 37,* 51–56.

Keefe, F. J., Caldwell, D. S., Martinez, S., Nunley, J., Beckham, J., & Williams, D. A. (1991). Analyzing pain in rheumatoid arthritis patients: Pain coping strategies in patients who have had knee replacement surgery. *Pain, 46,* 153–160.

Keefe, F. J., & Williams, D. A. (1990). A comparison of coping strategies in chronic pain patients in different age groups. *Journals of Gerontology, 45,* 161–165.

Keller, C. (1988). Psychological and physical variables as predictors of coping strategies. *Perceptual and Motor Skills, 67,* 95–100.

Kempen, G. I. J. M., Ormel, J., Brilman, E. I., & Relyveld, J. (1997). Adaptive responses among Dutch elderly: The impact of eight chronic medical conditions on health- related quality of life. *American Journal of Public Health, 87,* 38–44.

Kim, M., Nesselroade, J., & Featherman, D. (1996). The state component in self-reported world views and religious beliefs of older adults. The MacArthur Studies of Successful Aging. *Psychology and Aging, 11,* 396–407.

King, K. B., Reis, H. T., Porter, L. A., & Norsen, L. H. (1993). Social support and long-term recovery from coronary artery surgery: Effects on patients and spouses. *Health Psychology, 12,* 56–63.

King, K. B., Rowe, M. A., Kimble, L. P., & Zerwick, J. J. (1998). Optimism, coping and long-term recovery from coronary artery surgery in women. *Research in Nursing and Health, 21*(1), 15–26.

Knottnerus, J., et al. (1992). Chronic illness in the community and the concept of social prevalence. *Family Practice, 9,* 15–21.

Koenig, H. G. (1998). Depression in hospitalized older patients with congestive heart failure. *General Hospital Psychiatry, 20,* 29–43.

Koenig, H. G., et al. (1988). The use of religion and other emotion-regulating coping strategies among older adults. *Gerontologist, 28,* 303–310.

Koenig, H. G., Cohen, H. J., Blazer, D. G., & Pieper, C. (1992). Religious coping and depression among elderly, hospitalized medically ill men. *American Journal of Psychiatry, 149,* 1693–1700.

Kraditor, K. (2001). *Facts and trends: The assisted living sourcebook 2001.* Washington, DC: National Center for Assisted Living.

Kraemer, H. C. (1995). Statistical issues in assessing comorbidity. *Statistics in Medicine, 14,* 721–733.

Krause, N. A., Herzog, R., & Baker, E. (1992). Providing support to others and well-being in later life. *Journals of Gerontology: Psychological Sciences, 47,* P300–P311.

Kriegsman, D. M. W., Van Eijk, J. T. M., Penninx, B. W. J. H., Deeg, D. J. H., & Boeke, A. J. P. (1997). Does family support buffer the impact of specific chronic health conditions on mobility in community-dwelling elderly? *Disability and Rehabilitation, 19,* 71–83.

Krogh, V., Trevisan, M., Jossa. F., Bland, S., Jalowiec, A., Celentano, E., et al. (1992). Coping and blood pressure. *Journal of Human Hypertension, 6,* 65–70.

Krueger, R. A. (1998a). Analyzing and reporting focus group results. In D. L. Morgan & R. A. Krueger (Eds.), *The Focus Group Kit: Vol. 6.* Thousand Oaks, CA: Sage.

Krueger, R. A. (1998b). Developing questions for focus groups. In D. L. Morgan & R. A. Krueger (Eds.), *The Focus Group Kit: Vol. 3.* Thousand Oaks, CA: Sage.

Krumholz, H. M., Butler, J., Miller, J., Vaccarino, V., Williams, C. S., Mendes de Leon, et al. (1998). Prognostic importance of emotional support for elderly patients hospitalized with heart failure. *Cardiology, 97,* 958–964.

Kruse, A. (1987). Coping with chronic disease, dying and death: A contribution to competence in old age. *Comprehensive Gerontology, 1,* 1–11.

Kuhn, T. S. (1970). *The structure of scientific revolutions* (2nd ed.). Chicago: University of Chicago Press.

Lacasse, Y., Goldstein, R. S., & Guyatt, G. H. (1997). Respiratory rehabilitation in chronic obstructive pulmonary disease: Summary of a systematic overview of the literature. *Reviews in Clinical Gerontology, 7,* 327–347.

LaCroix, A. Z., Newton, K. M., Leveille, S. G., & Wallace J. (1997). Healthy aging: A women's issue. *Western Journal of Medicine, 67,* 220–232.

Laferriere, R. H., & Hamel Bissell, B. P. (1994). Successful aging of oldest old women in the Northeast Kingdom of Vermont. *IMAGE: Journal of Nursing Scholarship, 26,* 319–323.

Lakatos, I. (1977). The methodology of scientific research programmes. In J. W. G. Currie (Ed.), *Philosophical papers (Vol. 1).* Cambridge, UK: Cambridge University Press.

Landerville, P., Dube, M., Lalande, G., & Adain, M. (1994). Appraisal, coping, and depressive symptoms in older adults with reduced mobility. *Journal of Social Behavior and Personality, 9,* 269–286.

Landerville, P., & Vezina, J. (1994). Differences in appraisal and coping between elderly coronary artery disease patients high and low in depressive symptoms. *Journal of Mental Health: United Kingdom, 3*(1), 79–89.

Lanza, A. F., & Revenson, T. A. (1993). Social support interventions for rheumatoid arthritis patients: The cart before the horse. *Health Education Quarterly, 20,* 97–117.

La Rue, A. A., D'Elia, L. F., Clark, E. O., Spar, J. E., & Jarvik, L. F. (1986). Clinical tests of memory in dementia, depression, and healthy aging. *Journal of Psychology and Aging, 1,* 69–77.

Lasky, W. F. (1999, April 26). General Accounting Office Testimony [Available: online]. (Assisted Living Federation of America) www.alfa.org

Laudan, L. (1977). *Progress and its problems.* Los Angeles: University of California Press.

Lavery, J. F., & Clarke, V. A. (1996). Causal attributions, coping strategies, and adjustment to breast cancer. *Cancer Nursing, 19*(1), 20–28.

Lazarus, R. S. (1986). Stress and coping. In G. L. Maddox (Ed.), *Encyclopedia of aging* (pp. 647–649). New York: Springer.

Lazarus, R. S. (1999). *Stress and emotion: A new synthesis.* New York: Springer.

Lazarus, R. S. (2000). Toward better research on stress and coping. *American Psychologist, 55,* 665–673.

Lazarus, R. S., & Folkman, S. (1984). *Stress, appraisal and coping.* New York: Springer.

Lehr, U., & Kruse, A. (1992). Coping with health problems in old age: A longitudinal approach. *Aging Clinical and Experimental Research, 4,* 287–292.

Leigh, J. P., & Fries, J. F. (1992). Predictors of disability in a longitudinal sample of patients with rheumatoid arthritis. *Annals of Rheumatic Diseases, 51,* 581–587.

Lepore, S. J., & Evans, G. W. (1996). Coping with multiple stressors in the environment. In M. Zeidner & N. S. Endler (Eds.), *Handbook of coping* (pp. 350–377). New York: Wiley.

Lerner, M. J. (1992). *Is it coping or is it growth? A cognitive-affective model of contentment in the elderly: Life crises and experiences of loss in adulthood.* Hillsdale, NJ: Erlbaum.

Leventhal, H., Rabin, C., Leventhal, E. A., & Burns, E. (2001). Health risk behaviors and aging. In J. E. Birren & K. W. Schaie (Eds.), *Handbook of the psychology of aging* (5th ed., pp. 186–214). San Diego, CA: Academic Press.

Lewinsohn, P. M., Hoberman, H., Teri, L., & Hautzinger, M. (1985). An integrative theory of depression. In S. Reiss & R. R. Bootzin (Eds.), *Theoretical issues in behavior therapy* (pp. 331–359). New York: Academic.

Lin, C. C. (1998). Comparison of the effects of perceived self-efficacy on coping with chronic cancer pain and coping with chronic low back pain. *Clinical Journal of Pain, 14,* 303–310.

Lincoln, Y. S., & Guba, E. (1985). *Naturalistic inquiry.* Beverly Hills, CA: Sage.

Linn, B. S., Linn, M. W., & Gurel, L. (1968). Cumulative illness rating scale. *Journal of the American Geriatrics Society, 16,* 622–626.

Lipowski, Z. J. (1970). Physical illness, the individual and the coping process. *Psychiatry in Medicine, 1*(3), 91–102.

Litwin, H. (1998). The provision of informal support by elderly people residing in assisted living facilities. *Gerontologist, 38,* 239–246.

Lohman, T. G., Roche, A. F., & Martorell, R. (1988). *Anthropometric standardization reference manual.* Champaign, IL: Human Kinetics Books.

Lohr, M. J., Essex, M. J., & Klein, M. H. (1988). The relationships of coping responses to physical health status and life satisfaction among older women. *Journal of Gerontology, 43*, P54–P60.

Lopez, M. A., & Mermeistein, R. J. (1987). *Stress, coping and adaptation to chronic illness in hospitalized elderly: Predictors of treatment outcome.* Chicago: Rush University, Department of Psychology and Social Sciences.

Lorig, K. (1996). Chronic disease self-management: A model for tertiary prevention. *American Behavioral Scientist, 39*, 676–683.

Lorig, K. R., Sobel, D. S., Stewart, A. L., Brown, B. W., Bandura, A., Ritter, P., et al. (1999). Evidence suggesting that a chronic disease self-management program can improve health status while reducing hospitalization: A randomized trial. *Medical Care, 37*, 5–14.

Lyness, J. M., Duberstein, P. R., King, D. A., Cox, C., & Caine, E. D. (1999). Medical illness burden, trait neuroticism, and depression in older primary care patients. *American Journal of Psychiatry, 155*, 969–971.

Lyons, R. F., Sullivan, M. J. L., & Ritvo, P. G. (1995). The stressors of illness and disability. In R. F. Lyons, P. G. Ritvo, & J. C. Coyne (Eds.), *Relationships in chronic illness and disability* (pp. 19–37). Thousand Oaks, CA: Sage.

Maes, S., Leventhal, H., & de Ridder, D. T. (1996). Coping with chronic diseases. In M. Zeidner & N. Endler (Eds.), *Handbook of coping* (pp. 221–251). New York: John Wiley.

Mahat, G. (1997). Perceived stressors and coping strategies among individuals with rheumatoid arthritis. *Journal of Advanced Nursing, 25*, 1144–1150.

Manne, S. L., & Zautra, A. J. (1990). Couples coping with chronic illness: Women with rheumatoid arthritis and their healthy husbands. *Journal of Behavioral Medicine, 13*, 327–342.

Manton, K. G. (1988). A longitudinal study of functional change and mortality in the United States. *Journals of Gerontology: Social Sciences, 43*, S153–S161.

Manton, K. G., & Stallard, E. (1991). Cross-sectional estimates of active life expectancy for the U.S. elderly and oldest-old populations. *Journals of Gerontology: Social Sciences, 46*, S170–S182.

March, J. G., & Simon, H. A. (1958). *Organizations.* New York: Wiley.

Martin, P. (in press). Individual and social resources predicting well-being and functioning in the later years: Conceptual models, research, and practice. *Aging International.*

Martin, P., & Martin, M. (2002). Proximal and distal influences on development: The model of developmental adaptation. *Developmental Review, 22*, 78–96.

Martin, P., Poon, L. W., Clayton, G. M., Lee, H. S., Fulks, J. S., & Johnson, M. A. (1992). Personality, life events, and coping in the oldest-old. *International Journal of Aging and Human Development, 34* (1), 19–30.

Martin, P., Rott, C., Poon, L. W., Courtenay, B., & Lehr, U. (2001). A molecular view of coping behavior in older adults. *Journal of Aging and Health, 13*, 72–91.

Masoro, E. J. (2001). 'Successful aging': Useful or misleading concept? *Gerontologist, 41*, 415–418.

Mattlin, J. A., Wethington, E., & Kessler, R. C. (1990). Situational determinants of coping and coping effectiveness. *Journal of Health and Social Behavior, 13*, 103–122.

McCrae, R. R. (1999). Age differences and changes in the use of coping mechanisms. *Journal of Gerontology, 44,* 161–169.

McCulloch, B. J. (1990). The relationship of intergenerational reciprocity of aid to the morale of older parents: Equity and exchange theory comparisons. *Journals of Gerontology: Social Sciences, 45,* S150–S155.

McDermott, J. (1995). The first step. *Journal of the American Medical Association, 273,* 251–253.

McKee, P. L. (1982). *Philosophical foundations of gerontology.* New York: Human Sciences.

McKinlay, J. B., & McKinlay, S. M. (1977). The questionable contribution of medical measures to the decline of mortality in the United States in the twentieth century. *Milbank Memorial Fund Quarterly/Health and Society* (pp. 405–428).

Meeks, S., Carstensen, L. L., Tamsky, B. F., Wright, T. L., & Pellegrini, D. (1989). Age differences in coping: Does less mean worse? *International Journal of Aging and Human Development, 28,* 127–140.

Menard, S. (1991). *Longitudinal research.* Newbury Park, CA.: Sage University Papers.

Michael, S. R. (1996). Integrating chronic illness into one's life: A phenomenological inquiry. *Journal of Holistic Nursing, 14,* 251–267.

Miller, E., & Lewis, P. (1977). Recognition memory in elderly patients with depression and dementia: A signal detection analysis. *Journal of Abnormal Psychology, 86,* 84–86.

Miller, F. J. (1992). *Coping with chronic illness: Overcoming powerlessness* (2nd ed.). Philadelphia: Davis.

Molla, M. T., Wagener, D. K., & Madans, J. H. (2001). *Summary measures of population health methods for calculating healthy life expectancy: Healthy People Statistical Notes, No. 21.* Hyattsville, MD: National Center for Health Statistics.

Mollica, R. (2000). *State assisted living policy: 2000.* Portland, ME: National Academy for State Health Policy.

Montbriand, M. J., & Laing, G. P. (1991). Alternative health care as a control strategy. *Journal of Advanced Nursing, 16,* 325–332.

Moos, R. H. (Ed.). (1976). *Human adaptation: Coping with life crises.* Lexington, MA: Heath.

Moos, R. H. (Ed.). (1984). *Coping with physical illness: New directions* (Vol 2). New York: Plenum.

Moos, R. H., & Mertens, J. R. (1999). Patterns of diagnoses, comorbidities, and treatment in late-middle-aged and older affective disorder patients: Comparison of mental health and medical sectors. *Journal of the American Geriatrics Society, 44,* 682–688.

Morey, M. C., Cowper, P. A., Feussner, J. R., DiPasquale, R. C., Crowley, G. M., Kitzman. D. W., et al. (1989). Evaluation of a supervised exercise program in a geriatric population. *Journal of the American Geriatrics Society, 37,* 348–354.

Morgan, D. L. (1997). *Focus groups as qualitative research* (2nd ed., No. 16, Qualitative Research Methods Series). Thousand Oaks, CA: Sage.

Morgan, D. L. (1998a). The focus group guidebook. In D. L. Morgan & R. A. Krueger (Eds.), *The Focus Group Kit* (Vol. 1). Thousand Oaks, CA: Sage.

Morgan, D. L. (1998b). Planning focus groups. In D. L. Morgan & R. A. Krueger (Eds.), *The Focus Group Kit* (Vol. 2). Thousand Oaks, CA: Sage.

Morse, J. M., & Field, P. A. (1995). Qualitative research methods for health professionals. (2nd ed.). Thousand Oaks, CA: Sage.

Morse, J. M., & Johnson, J. L. (1991). Toward a theory of illness: The illness constellation model. In J. M. Morse & J. L. Johnson (Eds.), *The illness experience: Dimensions of suffering* (pp. 315–342). Newbury Park, CA: CA: Sage.

Murray, C. J. L., & Lopez, A. (1997). Regional patterns of disability-free life expectancy and disability-adjusted life expectancy: Global Burden of Disease Study. *Lancet, 349,* 1347–1352.

Murray, C. J. L., Salomon, J. A., & Mathers, C. (1999). *A critical examination of summary measures of population health. Global Programme on Evidence for Health Policy (GPE) Discussion Paper No. 2, Rev. 1.* World Health Organization.

Nagi, S. Z. (1976). An epidemiology of disability among adults in the United States. *Milbank Memorial Fund Quarterly,* 6, 493–508.

Narsavage, G. L. (1997). Promoting function in clients withchronic lung disease by increasing their perception of control. *Holistic Nursing Practice, 12,* 17–26.

National Center for Health Statistics. (2001). Mortality Data. [On-line]. Available: www.cdc.gov/nchs/about/major/dvs/mortdata.htm.

National Health Services Centre for Reviews and Dissemination (1996). *Undertaking systematic reviews of research on effectiveness: CRD guidelines for those carrying out or commissioning reviews. (CRD Report 4).* York, UK: National Health Services Centre for Reviews and Dissemination.

National Heart, Lung, and Blood Institute. (1998). *Clinical guidelines on the identification, evaluation, and treatment of overweight and obesity in adults.* Bethesda, MD: National Institutes of Health.

National Vital and Health Statistics Report. (1999). Centers for Disease Control and Prevention. [On-line]. Available: www.cdc.gov/nchs/nvss.htm

Neugarten, B., Havighurst, R., & Tobin, S. (1961). The measurement of life satisfaction. *Journal of Gerontology,* 134–143.

Newman, S. (1990). Coping with chronic illness. In P. Bennet, J. Weinman, & P. Spurgeon (Eds.), *Current developments in health psychology* (pp. 159–175). Chur, Switzerland: Harwood.

Niederehe, G. (1986). Depression and memory impairment in the aged. In L. W. Poon (Ed.), *Clinical memory assessment of older adults* (pp. 226–237). Washington, DC: American Psychological Association.

Norburn, J. E. K., Bernard, S. L., Konrad, T. R., & Woomert. A. (1995). Self-care and assistance from others in coping with functional status limitations among a national sample of older adults. *Journals of Gerontology: Series B: Psychological Sciences and Social Sciences, 50B,* S101–S109.

Nyklicek, I., Vingerhoets, A. J., Van Heck, G. L., & Van Limpt, M. C. (1998). Defensive coping in relation to casual blood pressure and self-reported daily hassles and life events. *Journal of Behavioral Medicine, 21*(2), 145–161.

Olshansky, S. J., & Wilkins, R. (1998). Introduction. Special issue: Policy implications of the measures and trends in health expectancy. *Journal of Aging and Health, 10*(2), 123–135.

Ormel, J., Kempen, G. I. J. M., Penninx, B. W. J. H., Brilman, E. I., Beekman, A. T. F., & Van Sonderen, E. (1997). Chronic medical conditions and mental health in older people: Disability and psychosocial resources mediate specific mental health effects. *Psychological Medicine, 27,* 1065–1077.

Ornish, D., Brown, S. E., Scherwitz, L. W., et al. (1990). Can lifestyle changes reverse coronary heart disease? *Lancet, 336,* 129–133.

Ostwald, S. K., Weiss Farnan, P., & Monson, T. (1990). The impact of health education on health status: An experimental program for elderly women in the community. *Journal of Community Health Nursing, 7,* 199–213.

Paffenbarger, R. S., Jr., Hyde, T. R., Wing, A. L., & Hsieh, C. (1986). Physical activity, all-cause mortality and longevity of college alumni. *New England Journal of Medicine, 314,* 605–613.

Palinkas, L. A., Wingard, D. L., & Barrett Connor, E. (1990). Chronic illness and symptoms in the elderly: A population-based study. *Journal of Clinical Epidemiology, 43,* 1131–1141.

Palmore, E. (1979). Predictors of successful aging. *Gerontologist, 19,* 427–431.

Parker, J., et al. (1988). Coping strategies in rheumatoid arthritis. *Journal of Rheumatology, 15,* 1376–1383.

Pearlin, L. I. (1991). The study of coping: An overview of problems and directions. In J. Eckenrode (Ed.), *The social context of coping* (pp. 261–276). New York: Plenum.

Pearlin, L. I., & Schooler, C. (1978). The structure of coping. *Journal of Health and Social Behavior, 19,* 2–22.

Pearlman, R. A., & Uhlmann, R. F. (1988). Quality of life in chronic diseases: Perceptions of elderly patients. *Journal of Gerontology, 43,* M25–M30.

Penninx, B. W., Beekman, A. T., Ormel, J., Kriegsman, D. M., Boeke, A. J., van Eijk, J. T., et al. (1996). Psychological status among elderly people with chronic health conditions: Does type of disease play a part? *Journal of Psychosomatic Research, 40,* 521–534.

Penninx, B. W. J. H., vanTilburg, T., Boeke, A. J. P., Deeg, D. J. H., Kriegsman, D. M. W., & vanEijk, J. T. M. (1998). Effects of social support and personal coping resources on depressive symptoms: Different for various chronic health conditions? *Health Psychology, 17,* 551–558.

Penninx, B. W. J. H., vanTilburg, T., Kriegsman, D. M. W., Deeg, D. J. H., Boeke, A. J. P., & van Eijk, J. T. M. (1997). Effects of social support and personal coping resources on mortality in older age: The longitudinal aging study in Amsterdam. *American Journal of Epidemiology, 146,* 510–519.

Petrie, A. D. (1990). A community-based health promotion project for persons with chronic respiratory disease. *Canadian Journal of Public Health, 81,* 310–312.

Pfeiffer, E. A. (1975). Short Portable Mental Status Questionnaire for the Assessment of Organic Brain Deficit in Elderly Patients. *Journal of the American Geriatrics Society, 23,* 433–441.

Phillips, D. (1987). *Philosophy, science, and social inquiry: Contemporary methodological controversies in social science and related applied fields of research.* New York: Pergamon.

Pollock, S. E. (1987). Adaptation to chronic illness. *Nursing Clinics of North America, 22,* 631–644.

Poon, L. W. (1985). Differences in human memory with aging: Nature, causes and clinical implications. In J. E. Birren & K. W. Shaie (Eds.), *Handbook of the psychology of aging* (pp. 427–455). New York: Van Nostrand Reinhold.

Poon, L. W. (1992). Toward an understanding of cognitive function in geriatric depression. [Special Research Award Issue]. *International Psychogeriatrics, 4,* 241–266.

Poon, L. W. (2001). Learning. In G. L. Maddox (Ed.), *The encyclopedia of aging: A comprehensive resource in gerontology and geriatrics* (3rd ed.). New York: Springer.

Popkin, S., Gallagher, D., Thompson, L. W., & Moore, M. (1982). Memory complaint and performance in normal and depressed older adults. *Experimental Aging Research, 8,* 141–145.

Powers, M. J., & Jalowiec, A. (1987). Profile of the well-controlled, well-adjusted hypertensive patient. *Nursing Research, 36,* 106–110.

Pruchno, R. A., Burant, C. J., & Peters, N. D. (1997). Understanding the well-being of care receivers. *Gerontologist, 37,* 102–109.

Putnam, R. D. (2000). *Bowling alone: The collapse and revival of American community.* New York: Simon & Schuster.

QSR International Pty. Ltd. (2000). *NVivo: Qualitative Data Analysis Program.* Version 1.2. Melbourne, Australia.

Quine, S., & Cameron, I. (1995). The use of focus groups with the disabled elderly. *Qualitative Health Research, 5,* 454–462.

Rader, M. C., & Vaughen, J. L. (1994). Management of the frail and deconditioned patient. *Southern Medical Journal, 87,* S61–S65.

Rakowski, W. (1984). Health psychology and later life: The differentiation of health and illness for the study of health-related behaviors. *Research on Aging, 6,* 593–620.

Rakowski, W., Pearlman, D. N., & Murphy, J. B. (1995). Successful aging: Psychosocial factors and implications for primary care geriatrics. In W. Reichel (Ed.), *Care of the elderly: Clinical aspects of aging* (4th ed., pp. 463–471). Baltimore: Williams & Wilkins.

Raleigh, E. D. (1992). Sources of hope in chronic illness. *Oncology Nursing Forum, 19,* 443–448.

Reed, P. G. (1995). A treatise on nursing knowledge development for the 21st century: Beyond postmodernism. *Advances in Nursing Science, 17*(3), 70–84.

Revenson, T. A., & Felton, B. J. (1989). Disability and coping as predictors of psychological adjustment to rheumatoid arthritis. *Journal of Consulting and Clinical Psychology, 57,* 344–348.

Revenson, T. A., Woliman, C. A., & Felton, B. J. (1983). Social supports as stress buffers for adult cancer patients. *Psychosomatic Medicine, 45,* 321–331.

Revicki, D. A., & Mitchell, J. P. (1990). Strain, social support, and mental health in rural elderly individuals. *Journal of Gerontology, 45,* S267–S274.

Rijken, P. M., & Dekker, J. (1998). Clinical experience of rehabilitation therapists with chronic health conditions: A quantitative approach. *Clinical Rehabilitation, 2,* 143–150.

Riley, M. W. (1998). Letters to the Editor. *Gerontologist, 38,* 151.

Riley, M. W., Foner, A., & Waring, J. (1988). Sociology of age. In N. Smelser, (Ed.), *Handbook of sociology* (pp. 143–290). Newbury Park, CA: Sage.

Riley, M. W., Huber, B. J., & Hess, B. (Eds.). (1988). *Social structures and human lives*. Newbury Park, CA: Sage.

Riley, M. W., & Riley, J. W. (1990). Structural lag: Past and future. In M. W. Riley, R. L. Kahn, & A. Foner (Eds.), *Age and structural lag* (pp.15–36). New York: Wiley.

Roberson, M. H. (1992). The meaning of compliance: Patient perspectives. *Qualitative Health Research, 2*, 7–26.

Roberto, K.A. (1989). *Stress and adaptation patterns of older osteoporotic women*. New York: Haworth.

Roberto, K. A. (1992). Coping strategies of older women with hip fractures: Resources and outcomes. *Journal of Gerontology, 47*(1), 21–26.

Roberts, J., Browne, G. B., Streiner, D., Gafni, A., Pallister, R., Hoxby, H., et al. (1995). Problem-solving counseling or phone-call support for outpatients with chronic illness: Effective for whom? *Canadian Journal of Nursing Research, 27*, 111–137.

Roberts, R. E., Kaplan, G. A., Shema, S. J., & Strawbridge, W. J. (1997). Does growing old increase the risk for depression? *American Journal of Psychiatry, 154*, 1384–1390.

Robine, J. M. (2000). Setting up of a coherent set of health expectancies for the European Union. Euro-REVES II.

Robinson, C. A. (1993). Managing life with a chronic condition: The story of normalization. *Qualitative Health Research, 3*, 6–28.

Rodin, J., & McAvay, G. (1992). Determinants of change in perceived health in a longitudinal study of older adults. *Journal of Gerontology: Psychological Science, 47*, P373–P384.

Rolfe, G. (1999). The pleasure of the bottomless: Postmodernism, chaos, and paradigm shifts. *Nurse Education Today, 19*, 668–672.

Rook, K. S. (1987). Reciprocity of social exchange and social satisfaction among older women. *Journal of Personality and Social Psychology, 52*, 145–154.

Rook, K. S., & Dooley, D. (1985). Applying social support research: Theoretical problems and future directions. *Journal of Social Issues, 41*, 5–28.

Roos, N., & Havens, B. (1991). Predictors of successful aging: A twelve-year study of Manitoba elderly. *American Journal of Public Health, 81*, 63–68.

Rosenberg, S. J., Peterson, R. A., & Hayes, J. R. (1987). Coping behaviors among depressed and non-depressed medical inpatients. *Journal of Psychosomatic Research, 31*, 653–658.

Rosenstock, I. M., Strecher, V. J., & Becker, M. (1988). Social learning theory and the health belief model. *Health Education Quarterly, 15*, 175–183.

Rosow, I., & Breslau, N. (1966). A Guttman Health Scale for the Aged. *Journal of Gerontology, 21*, 556–559.

Roter, D. L., Hall, J. A., Merisca, R., Nordstrom, B., Cretin, D., & Svarstad, B. (1998). Effectiveness of interventions to improve patient compliance: A meta-analysis. *Medical Care, 36*, 1138–1161.

Roth, S., & Cohen, L. J. (1986). Approach, avoidance and coping with stress. *American Psychologist, 41*, 813–819.

Rothenberg, B. M., Mooney, C., Curtis, L., Andresen, E. E., Rothenberg, B. E., &

Zimmer, J. G. (Eds.). (1997). Measures of severity of illness and comorbidity. In *Assessing the health status of older adults*. New York: Springer.

Rowe, J. W., & Kahn, R. L. (1987). Human aging: Usual and successful. *Science, 237,* 143–149.

Rowe, J. W., & Kahn, R. L. (1997). Successful aging. *Gerontologist, 37,* 433–480.

Rowe, J. W., & Kahn, R. L. (1998). *Successful aging: The MacArthur Foundation Study.* New York: Pantheon.

Ruberman, W., Weinblatt, E., Goldberg, J. D., & Chaudhary, B. S. (1984). Psychosocial influences on mortality after myocardial infarction. *New England Journal of Medicine, 311,* 552–559.

Rybarczyk, B., DeMarco, G., DelaCruz, M., & Lapidos, S. (1999). Comparing mind-body wellness interventions for older adults with chronic illness: Classroom versus home instruction. *Behavioral Medicine, 24,* 181–190.

Ryff, C. (1989). Beyond Ponce de Leon and life satisfaction: New directions in quest of successful aging. *International Journal of Behavioral Development, 12,* 35–55.

Saito, Y., Crimmins, E. M., & Hayward, M. D. (1999). *Health expectancy: An overview.* (Nihon University Research Paper Series, No. 67). Tokyo: Nihon University.

Sanders, B. S. (1964). Measuring community health levels. *American Journal of Public Health, 54,* 1063–1070.

Sarason, B. R., Sarason, I. G., & Pierce, G. R. (1990). Traditional views of social support and their impact on assessment. In B. R. Sarason, I. G. Sarason, & G. R. Pierce (Eds.), *Social support: An interactional view* (pp. 7–25). New York: Wiley.

Schaefer, C., Coyne, J. C., & Lazarus, R. S. (1981). The health-related functions of social support. *Journal of Behavioral Medicine, 4,* 430–435.

Schaie, K. W., & Hofer, S. M. (2001). Longitudinal studies in aging research. In J. E. Birren & K. W. Schaie (Eds.), *Handbook of the psychology of aging* (5th ed., pp. 53–77). San Diego: Academic.

Schaie, K. W., & Willis, S. L. (1986). Can adult intellectual decline be reversed? *Developmental Psychology, 22,* 223–232.

Scharloo, M., Kaptein, A. A., Weinman, J., Hazes, J. M., Willems, L., Bergman, W., et al. (1998). Illness perceptions, coping and functioning in patients with rheumatoid arthritis, chronic obstructive pulmonary disease, and psoriasis. *Journal of Psychosomatic Research, 44,* 573–585.

Scheier, M. F., Carver, C. S., & Bridges, M. W. (1994). Distinguishing optimism from neuroticism (and trait anxiety, self-mastery, and self-esteem): A re-evaluation of the Life Orientation Test. *Journal of Personality and Social Psychology, 67,* 1063–1078.

Schellevis, F. G., van der Velden, J., van de Lisdonk, E., van Eijk, J. T., & van Weel, C. (1993). Comorbidity of chronic health conditions in general practice. *Journal of Clinical Epidemiology, 46,* 469–473.

Schmidt, R. M. (1994). Healthy aging into the 21st century. *Contemporary Gerontology, 1,* 3–6.

Schoeni, R. F., Freedman, V. A., & Wallace, R. B. (2001). Persistent, consistent, widespread, and robust? Another look at trends in old-age disability. *Journal of Gerontology, 56,* S206–S218.

Schrag, C. O. (1997). *The self after postmodernity.* New Haven, CT: Yale University Press.

Schreurs, K., & de Ridder, D. (1997). Integration of coping and social support perspectives: Implications for the study of adaptation to chronic diseases. *Clinical Psychology Review, 17,* 89–112.

Schussler, G. (1999). Coping strategies and individual meanings of illness. *Social Science Medicine, 34,* 427–432.

Scott, B., Lindberg, P., Melin, L., & Lyttkens, L. (1994). Control and dispositional style among the hearing-impaired in communication situations. *Audiology, 33,* 177–184.

Scriven, M. (1969). *The legacy of logical positivism.* Baltimore: Johns Hopkins Press.

Seeman, T. E. (1994). Successful aging: Reconceptualizing the aging process from a more positive perspective. *Facts and Research in Gerontology, 8,* 3–15.

Seeman, T. E., Berkman, L. F., Blazer, D., & Rowe, J. (1994). Social ties and support and neuroendocrine function: The MacArthur Studies of Successful Aging. *Annals of Behavioral Medicine, 16,* 95–106.

Seeman, T. E., Berkman, L. F., Charpentier, P., Blazer, D., Albert, M., & Tinetti, M. (1995). Behavioral and psychosocial predictors of physical performance: The MacArthur Studies of Successful Aging. *Journal of Gerontology: Medical Science, 50A,* M177–M183.

Seeman, T. E., Berkman, L. F., Kohout, F., et al. (1993). Intercommunity variation in the association between social ties and mortality in the elderly: A comparative analysis of three communities. *Annals of Epidemiology, 3,* 325–335.

Seeman, T. E., Charpentier, P. A., Berkman, L. F., Tinetti, M. E., Guralnik, J. M., Albert, M. S., et al. (1994). Predicting changes in physical performance in a high functioning elderly cohort: The MacArthur Studies of Successful Aging. *Journal of Gerontology: Medical Science, 49,* M97–M108.

Seeman, T. E., Levy-Storms, L., Singer, B., & Ryff, C. (in press). Psychosocial factors and the development of allostatic load. *Psychosomatic Medicine.*

Seeman, T. E., Rodin, J., & Albert, M. (1993). Self-efficacy and cognitive performance in high-functioning older individuals: The MacArthur Studies of Successful Aging. *Journal of Aging and Health, 5,* 455–474.

Seeman, T. E., Singer, B., Horwitz, R., & McEwen, B. S. (1997). The price of adaptation: Allostatic load and its health consequences: The MacArthur Studies of Successful Aging. *Archives of Internal Medicine, 157,* 2259–2268.

Shaul, M. P. (1995). From early twinges to mastery: The process of adjustment in living with rheumatoid arthritis. *Arthritis Care Research, 8,* 290–297.

Sherbourne, C. D., Hays, R. D., & Wells, K. B. (1995). Personal and psychosocial risk factors for physical and mental health outcomes and course of depression among depressed patients. *Journal of Consulting and Clinical Psychology, 63,* 345–355.

Sherbourne, C. D., Meredith. L. S., Rogers, W., & Ware, J. E. J. (1992). Social support and stressful life events: Age differences in their effects on health-related quality of life among the chronically ill. *Quality of Life Research, 1,* 235–246.

Shin, Y. H. (1999). The effects of a walking exercise program on physical function and emotional state of elderly Korean women. *Public Health Nursing, 16,* 146–154.

Shumaker, S. A., & Brownell, A. (1984). Towards a theory of social support: Closing conceptual gaps. *Journal of Social Issues, 40,* 11–36.

Sidell, N. L. (1997). Adult adjustment to chronic illness: A review of the literature. *Health and Social Work, 22,* 5–11.

Silver, R. L., & Wortman, C. (1980). Coping with undesirable life events. In J. Garber & M. E. P. Seligman (Eds.), *Human helplessness* (pp. 279–340). New York: Academic Press.

Smith, J., & Couch, R. H. (1990). Adjustment services and aging. *Vocational Evaluation and Work Adjustment Bulletin, 23,* 133–138.

Smyer, M. A. (1995). Formal support in later life: Lessons for prevention. In L. A. Bond, S. J. Cutler, & A. Grams (Eds.), *Promoting successful and productive aging* (pp. 186–202). Thousand Oaks, CA: Sage.

Somerfield, M. R., & McCrae. R. R. (2000). Stress and coping research: Methodological challenges, theoretical advances, and clinical applications. *American Psychologist, 55,* 620–625.

Spector, W. D., Reschovsky, J. D., & Cohen, J. W. (1996). Appropriate placement of nursing-home residents in lower levels of care. *Milbank Quarterly, 74,* 139–160.

Sperling, U. (2000). Allgemeine und spezifiscihe Reaktionsformen in unterschiedlichen Bereichen des täglichen Lebens [General and specific coping reactions in differing domains of daily life]. In P. Martin, K. U. Ettrich, U. Lehr, D. Roether, M. Martin, & A. Fischer-Cyrulies (Eds.), *Aspekte der entwicklung im mittleren und höheren lebensalter: Ergebnisse der Interdisziplinären Längsschnittstudie des Erwachsenenalters (ILSE)* (pp. 83–97). Darmstadt, Germany: Steinkopff.

Spiegel, D. (1999). A 43–year-old woman coping with cancer. *Journal of the American Medical Association, 282,* 371–378.

Steffens, D. C., O'Connor, C. M., Jiang, W. J., Pieper, C., Kuchibhatla, M. N., Arias, R. M., et al. (1999). The effect of major depression on functional status in patients with coronary artery disease. *Journal of the American Geriatrics Society, 47,* 319–322.

Stephens, M. A., Kinney, J. M., Norris, V. K., & Ritchie, S. W. (1987). Social patients. *Psychology and Aging, 2,* 125–129.

Stewart, A. L., Greenfield, S., Hays, R. D., Wells, K. B., Rogers, W. H., Berry, S. D., et al. (1989). Functional status and well-being of patients with chronic conditions: Results from the Medical Outcomes Study. *Journal of the American Medical Association, 262,* 907–913.

Stewart, A. L., Hays, R. D., Wells, K. B., Rogers, W. H., Spritzer, K. L., & Greenfield, S. (1994). Long-term functioning and well-being outcomes associated with physical activity and exercise in patients with chronic conditions in the Medical Outcomes Study. *Journal of Clinical Epidemiology, 47,* 719–730.

Strack, S., & Feifel, H. (1996). Age differences, coping, and the adult life span. In M. Zeidner & N. S. Endler (Eds.), *Handbook of coping* (pp. 485–501). New York: Wiley.

Strain, L. A. (1996). Lay explanations of chronic illness in later life. *Journal of Aging and Health, 8,* 3–26.

Strauss, A. L. & Glasser, B. G. (1975). *Chronic illness and the quality of life*. St. Louis, MO: Mosby.

Strauss, G. (1972.) Is there a blue-collar revolt against work? In J. O'Toole (Ed.), *Work and the quality of life*. Cambridge: Massachusetts Institute of Technology Press.

Strawbridge, W. J., Cohen, R. D., Kurata, J., & Kaplan, G. A. (2000). Re: Physical activity and cardiovascular disease risk in middle-aged and older women. *American Journal of Epidemiology 151*, 736–737.

Strawbridge, W. J., Cohen, R. D., Shema, S. J., & Kaplan, G. K. (1996). Successful aging: Predictors and associated activities. *American Journal of Epidemiology, 144*, 135–141.

Strawbridge, W. J., Wallhagen, M. I., Shema, S. J., & Kaplan, G. A. (2000). Negative consequences of hearing impairment in old age: A longitudinal analysis. *Gerontologist, 40*, 320–326.

Sugisawa, H., Liang, J., & Liu, X. (1994). Social networks, social support, and mortality among older people in Japan. *Journal of Gerontology, 49*, S3–S13.

Sullivan, D. F. (1971). A single index of mortality and morbidity. *HSMHA Health Reports. 86*, 347–354.

Suls, J., & Fletcher, B. (1985). The relative efficacy of avoidant and nonavoidant coping strategies: A meta analysis. *Health Psychology, 4*, 249–288.

Sweeney, J. A., Wetzler, S., Stokes, P., & Kocsis, J. (1989). Cognitive functioning in depression. *Journal of Clinical Psychology, 45*, 836–842.

Taylor, H. L., Jacobs, D. R., Schucker, J., Knudson, J., Leon, A. S., & Debacker, G. (1978). A questionnaire for the assessment of leisure-time physical activity. *Journal of Chronic Diseases, 31*, 741–755.

Tennen, H., Affleck, G., Armeli, S., & Carney, M. A. (2000). A daily process approach to coping: Linking theory, research, and practice. *American Psychologist, 55*, 626–636.

Thornbury, K. M. (1982). Coping: Implications for health practitioners. *Patient Counselor. Health Education, 4*(1), 3–9.

Unger, J., McAvay, G., Bruce, M., Berkman, L. F., & Seeman, T. E. (1999). Variation in the impact of social network characteristics on physical functioning in elderly persons. The MacArthur Studies of Successful Aging. *Journal of Gerontology: Social Science, 54B*, S245–S252.

U.S. Bureau of the Census. (1996). *Current population reports. Series P25–1130. Population projections of the United States by age, sex, race, and Hispanic origin: 1995 to 2050*. Washington, DC: U.S. Government Printing Office.

U.S. Bureau of the Census. (1997). *Listing and coverage manual for field representatives*. Washington, DC: U.S. Government Printing Office.

U.S. Department of Health and Human Services. (1998, November). *Tracking healthy people 2000*. Washington, DC: U.S. Government Printing Office.

Vaillant, G. E. (1994). "Successful aging" and psychosocial well-being: Evidence from a 45–year study. In E. H. Thompson (Ed.), *Older men's lives* (pp. 22–41). Thousand Oaks, CA: Sage.

Vaillant, G. E. (2000). Adaptive mental mechanisms: Their role in a positive psychology. *American Psychologist, 55*, 89–98.

Valentine-Garzon, M. A., Maynard, M., & Selznick, S. Z. (1992). ROM Dance Program effects on frail elderly women in an adult day-care center. *Physical and Occupational Therapy in Geriatrics, 11,* 633–683.

Van den Akker, M., Buntinx, F., & Knottnerus, J. A. (1996). Comorbidity or multimorbidity: What's in a name? A review of the literature. *European Journal of General Practice, 2,* 65–70.

Van den Akker, M., Buntinx, F., Metsemakers, J. F., Roos, S., & Knottnerus, J. A. (1998). Multimorbidity in general practice: Prevalence, incidence, and determinants of co-occurring chronic and recurrent diseases. *Journal of Clinical Epidemiology, 51,* 367–375.

Vandelisdonk, E., Furer, J. W., Kroonen, A. P. M., & Marijnissen, A. G. M. M. (1992). Cataract functioning and comorbidity: A cross-sectional study in family practice. *Family Practice, 9,* 279–283.

Verbrugge, L., & Jette, A. (1994). The disablement process. *Social Science and Medicine, 38* (1), 1–14.

Verbrugge, L. M., Gates, D. M., & Ike, R. W. (1991). Risk factors for disability among U.S. adults with arthritis. *Journal of Clinical Epidemiology, 44,* 167–182.

Verbrugge, L. M., Lepkowski, J. M., & Imanaka, Y. (1989). Comorbidity and its impact on disability. *Milbank Quarterly, 67,* 450–484.

Verbrugge, L. M., Lepkowski, J. M., & Konkol, L. L. (1991). Levels of disability among U.S. adults with arthritis. *Journal of Gerontology, 46,* S71–S83.

Verbrugge, L. M., & Patrick, D. L. (1995). Seven chronic conditions: Their impact on U.S. adults' activity levels and use of medical services. *American Journal of Public Health, 85,* 173–182.

Viney, L. L., & Westbrook, M. T. (1986). Is there a pattern of psychological reactions to chronic illness which is associated with death? *Journal of Death and Dying, 17,* 169–181.

Vitiello, M. V., Prinz, P. N., Poon, L. W., & Williams, D. E. (1990, November). *Memory impairment in the elderly is associated with validated memory compliant but not with major depressive disorder.* Abstract presented at the 43rd Annual Meeting of the Gerontological Society of America, Boston, MA.

Wahl, H-W., Oswald, F., & Zimprich, D. (1999). Everyday competence in visually impaired older adults: A case for person-environment perspectives. *Gerontologist, 39,* 140–149.

Wallhagen, M. I., Strawbridge, W. J., Cohen, R. D., & Kaplan, G. A. (1997). Increasing prevalence of hearing impairment and associated risk factors over three decades of the Alameda County Study. *American Journal of Public Health, 87,* 440–442.

Wallhagen, M. I., Strawbridge, W. J., & Kaplan, G.A. (2001). Five-year impact of hearing impairment on physical functioning, mental health, and social relationships. *British Society of Audiology News, 32,* 9–11.

Wallhagen, M. I., Strawbridge, W. J., Shema, S. J., Kurata, J., & Kaplan, G. A. (2001). Comparative impact of hearing and vision impairment on subsequent functioning. *Journal of the American Geriatrics Society, 49,* 1101–1104.

Walker, B. L., Nail, L. M., Larsen, L., Magill, J., & Schwartz, A. (1996). Concerns, affect and cognitive disruption following completion of radiation treatment for localized breast or prostate cancer. *Oncology Nursing Forum, 23,* 1181–1187.

Walker, L., & Avant, K. (1995). *Strategies for theory construction in nursing* (3rd ed.). Norwalk, CT: Appleton & Lange.

Walker, M. K., Whincup, P. H., Shaper, G., Lennon, L. T., & Thomason, A.G. (1998). Validation of patient recall of doctor-diagnosed heart attack and stroke: A postal questionnaire and record review comparison. *American Journal of Epidemiology, 148,* 355–361.

Ward, M. M., & Leigh, J. P. (1993). Marital status and the progression of functional disaiblitiy in patients with rheumatoid arthritis. *Arthritis and Rheumatism, 36,* 581–588.

Welin, L., Larsson, B., Svardsudd, K., Tibbins, B., & Tibbins, G. (1992). Social network and activities in relation to mortality from cardiovascular diseases, cancer and other causes: A 12–year follow-up of the study of men born in 1913 and 1923. *Journal of Epidemiological Community Health, 46,* 127–132.

Wentowski, G. (1981). Reciprocity and the coping strategies of older people: Cultural dimensions of network building. *Gerontologist, 21,* 600–609.

Whall, A., & Hicks, F. (2002). The unrecognized paradigm shift within nursing. *Nursing Outlook, 50*(2), 72–76.

White, N. E., Richter, J. M., & Fry, C. (1992). Coping, social support, and adaptation to chronic illness. *Western Journal of Nursing Research, 14,* 211–224.

Wilcox, V. L., Kasi, S. V., & Berkman, L. F. (1994). Social support and physical disability in older people after hospitalization: A prospective study. *Health Psychology, 13,* 170–179.

Wilkie, D. J., & Keefe, F. J. (1991). Coping strategies of patients with lung cancer related pain. *Clinical Journal of Pain, 7,* 292–299.

Williams, R. H., & Wirths, C. G. (1965). *Lives through the years: Styles of life and successful aging.* New York: Atherton.

Woller, W., Kruse, J., Alberti, L., Kraut, D., Richter, B., Worth, H., et al. (1992). Affektiv-kognitive anfallsverarbeitung und krankheitsverhalten bei patienten mit asthma bronchiale [Coping with attacks and illness behavior in patients with bronichial asthma]. *Psychotherapie, Psychosomatik und Medizinische Psychologie, 42,* 63–70.

Woodard, G. M., Berry, M. J., Rejeski, W. J., Ribisi, P. M., & Miller, H. S. (1994). Exercise training in patients with cardiovascular disease and coexistent knee arthritis. *Journal of Cardiopulmonary Rehabilitation, 14,* 255–261.

World Health Organization. (1999). *The World Health report 1999: Making a difference.* Geneva, Switzerland: Author.

Yasuda, N., Zimmerman, S. I., Hawkes, W., Fredman, L., Hebel, J. R., & Magaziner, J. (1997). Relation of social network characteristics to 5–year mortality among young-old versus old-old white women in an urban community. *American Journal of Epidemiology, 145,* 516–523.

Young, W. (1994). Incorporating severity of illness and comorbidity in case-mix measurement. *Health Care Financing Review, 9,* 23–31.

Zeidner, M., & Saklofske, D. (1996). Adaptive and maladaptive coping. In M. Zeidner & N. S. Endler (Eds.), *Handbook of coping* (pp. 505–531). New York: Wiley.

Index

Index

Activities, 106
  of daily living, 106
  in old age, 7, 15–16
Acute bouts, 196
Adaptation, 171–172
  coping, 216
  developmental, 217
  successful, 217
Additive effect
  comorbidity, 169
Administrators
  assisted living, 48–49
Affective, 160
  cardiovascular disease influences,
    156, 157
  and cognitive, 160
    cardiovascular disease, 157
    coping strategy, 140–142
  cognitive and physical, 161–162
    cardiovascular disease, 158
    coping strategy, 144
  coping strategy, 139
Aggregative, 171
Aging
  changing our thinking, 109–110
  healthy, 2, 26
  MacArthur Studies of Successful
    Aging, 2, 83–103
  managing everyday life, 185
  plasticity of, 26
  productive, 2, 26
  self-rated successful aging
    correlates and predictors, 1–23
  in terms of reciprocity
    Rakowski, 227
  usual
    and successful aging, 26

Aging successfully, *see also* Successful
    aging
  Baltes and Baltes, 3
  premises, 27–29
  Schmidt's approach, 3
  self-ratings, 12–15
  ways to succeed, 39
Aging well, 2
Alameda County Study, 5
Analytic strategies
  of successful aging, 11–12
Ann Landers newspaper column, 116
Applying effective interventions, 175–
    177
Appraisal
  hypothesized coping model, 214
Arthritis, 84, 165
Assessment of effectiveness, 206
Assimilative, 171
Assisted living
  administrators, 48–49
  definition, 31–32
  economics, 50
  infrastructure, 49
  ladder ratings, 40, 41, 50–51, 51–52
  Likert-type indices, 34–35, 41, 51–52
  little things, 48–49, 51
  perceptions, 51
  reciprocity, 34–35
  resident
    characteristics, 36–38
    driving, 52
    interviews, 33–34
  responses, 41
  self-anchored ladder rating scale, 34–
    35
  Senior Olympics, 53

Assisted living (*continued*)
  settings
    reciprocity among older adults,
      25–53
  social network characteristics, 53
  staff, 48–49
    characteristics, 38
    interviews, 36
  subjective anchors, 52–53
Asthma
  coping responses, 211
Autonomy
  coping strategy, 136–139
Avoidance, 207
  coping, 123

Baltes and Baltes' conceptualization
    successful aging, 3, 114
Baltes selection-optimization-
    compensation model, 67
Barriers to understanding, 119–121
Behavioral factors, 88
Behavioral theory of stress, 122
Bivariate analysis
  managing everyday life, 185
Bivariate correlations
  between successful aging and
    reciprocity, 42–43
Bottomless swamp, 223

Cancer
  coping responses, 211
  functioning, 102
Cardiovascular disease, 164
  coping strategies, 155–159
    affective, 156–157
    affective, cognitive and physical,
      158
    affective and cognitive, 157
    cognitive and physical, 157–158
    physical, 156
  functioning, 156
  individual factors affecting coping,
    158
  social support for coping, 158
Cartesian mind–body dichotomy, 221
Causality, 168
Causes, 122
Challenges
  external, 198
  feeling challenged, 197–198
  internal, 197
Changing course, 203
Checking on myself, 205

Chronic conditions, 181
  list of 11, 183
  prevalence, 86
Chronic disease
  deaths, 209
  and disability, 70–82
  individual factors affecting coping,
    129
Chronic health conditions
  age differences in coping, 125–126
  coping, 151–179
  coping strategies, 135–144
  coping with, 122
  impact, 116–117
Chronic obstructive pulmonary disease
    (COPD), 164–165
Chronic stress
  hypothesized coping model, 214
Clinical practice
  recommendations, 174–175
Clustering, 168
Coexisting health problems, 116
Cognitive
  cardiovascular disease, 156, 157
  coping behaviors
    diseases, 159–160
  coping strategy, 135
Cognitive, affective, and physical, 161–
    162
  cardiovascular disease, 158
  coping strategy, 144
Cognitive and affective, 160
  cardiovascular disease, 157
  coping strategy, 140–142
Cognitive and physical, 160–161
  cardiovascular disease, 157–158
  coping strategy, 142–144
Cognitive-behavioral theory of stress,
    122
Cognitive coping, 122
  mechanisms, 216
Comorbidity, 181
  additive effect, 169
  assessment, 120
  concerns, 191–193
  coping with, 116–151
    gender, 127–128
    personality, 127–128
  definitions, 119–121
  ecology of coping, 193–204
  effects, 164–166
  modifying effect, 169–170
  multiplicative effect, 169
  Poon's thoughts on, 227

quality of life, 121
theory on effects of coping, 168–173
Conceptual issues, 212
Concurrence, 168
Consequences, 122
  intended and unintended, 55–69
Context stripping perspective, 223
Continuing on, 202, 205
Controllability, 122
COPD, 164–165
Coping
  adaptation, 216
  age differences
    chronic health conditions, 125–126
  avoidance, 123
  chronic disease, 129
  chronic health conditions, 122, 151–179
  comorbidity, 116–151, 168–173
    ecology of, 193–204
    gender, 127–128
    personality, 127–128
  definitions, 119–122
  depression, 166
  dying and death, 134
  effective
    age a risk factor, 123–124
  health problems
    life and nonlife-threatening, 133–134
  hypothesized model, 214
  individual factors affecting
    cardiovascular disease, 158
  literature, 210
  models, 122
    appraisal, 214
  multiple chronic health conditions,
    209–219
  with pain, 166–167
    strategies, 167
  problem-based, 207
  problem-focused, 123
  researchers
    self-criticism, 145–146
  research issues
    solutions, 148–149
  social support, 162–164
    for cardiovascular disease, 158
  successful
    social context, 128–130
  theory on effects of, 168–173
  ways, 122–123
Coping for life, 130–134
Coping over time course
  disease, 132–133

Coping responses
  asthma, 211
  cancer, 211
  diabetes, 211
  effective, 215–216
  effective evaluation, 215
  Margaret Wallhagen thoughts on,
    216
Coping strategies
  affective, 139
  affective, cognitive and physical, 144
  affective and cognitive, 140–142
  autonomy, 136–139
  cardiovascular disease, 155–159
  chronic health conditions, 135–144
  cognitive, 135
    diseases, 159–160
  cognitive, affective, and physical, 144
  cognitive and affective, 140–142
  cognitive and physical, 142–144
  counteractive effect, 170
  disease categories, 153–164
  interactive effect, 170
  pain, 167
Coping studies
  strengths and weaknesses, 146–147
Counteractive effect
  coping strategies, 170
Crimmins, Eileen, 104–106
Crimmins study
  chronic illness and disability, 114
Crossover, 173

Death
  coping with, 134
  of spouse, 210
Demographic variables, 11
Denial, 216
Denial model, 172
Depression, 131–132
  coping relationship, 166
Descriptive baseline data, 92–93
Developmental adaptation, 217
Diabetes
  coping responses, 211
Diabetes mellitus, 164
Disability
  and chronic disease, 70–82
Disability-free life expectancy, 106
Disease, see also specific types
  coping over time course, 132–133
  functioning, 101
  life with and without, 77–78
  symptoms, 130–134

Disease-specific, 168
Divorce, 210
Driving
    assisted living, 52
Dying
    coping with, 134
    of spouse, 210
Dynamism of changing lives, 67
Dynamism of structural change, 67

Economics
    assisted living, 50
    neighborhood and financial
        problems, 10
Education, 87–88, 124–127, 175–176
Effective coping
    age a risk factor, 123–124
    responses, 215–216
        evaluation, 215
Effective interventions, 175–177
Effectiveness
    assessment of, 206
Emic perspective, 182
Emotion-focused or cognitive strategies,
    207
Emotional support
    functioning, 101
Empowerment, 176–177
Encountering chronicity, 195–197
EPESE, 26
Established Populations for
    Epidemiologic Studies of the
    Elderly (EPESE), 26
Ethnicity, 11, 87–88
Expectations for the future, 206
External challenges, 198
External demands
    hypothesized coping model, 214

Feeling challenged, 197–198
Fighting a battle, 193
Financial problems, 10
Flare-ups, 195
Focus groups, 186–187
    format, 189–190
    methods
        living with multiple chronic
            illnesses, 190
Folkman and Lazarus model, 205
Four Ds (disease, disability, dementia,
    and death), 2
Fractures
    functioning, 102
Functional capability, 107
Functional disability

risks for, 83–84
Functioning
    cardiovascular disease influences, 156
    social and psychological factors, 100

Gender
    coping with comorbidity, 127–128
    differences
        health research, 107
        managing everyday life, 185
Give in, 207
Giving in to it, 199–200
Group dynamics
    living with multiple chronic illnesses,
        190
Groups, see Focus groups

Handling it a bit longer, 202
Health behaviors, 7, 94
Health care professionals
    educating, 177–178
Health conditions, see also specific type
    alleviate, 123
    coexisting, 116
    coping, 122, 151–179
        age differences in, 125–126
        strategies, 135–144
    impact, 116–117
    multiple, 118
    multiple chronic
        coping with, 209–219
        managing, 181–208
    nonlife-threatening
        coping, 133–134
Health expectancy, 104–115, 227
    across populations
        measuring, 107–109
    definition, 105–106
    impact, 70–82
Health problems, see Health conditions
Health promotion, 2
Health status, 112
    measures, 90
Healthy aging, 2, 26
Healthy life, 105
Hearing impairment, 10, 22, 165–166
Hypothesized coping model, 214
    appraisal, 214

Identification, 122
Implications
    Staying in Control, 204
Individual factors affecting coping
    cardiovascular disease, 158
Infrastructure

assisted living, 49
Institutional populations, 108
Intended consequences, 55–69
Interactive effect
    coping strategies, 170
Internal challenges, 197
Internal demands
    hypothesized coping model, 214
Interpersonal efficacy beliefs, 89
Interventions
    applying effective, 175–177
    therapeutic, 177
Introspective processes
    reflecting on self, 202

Joy in Texas, 116–120
Just the way it is, 205
Just too much, 211

Kahn, Robert, 1, 110
    coping literature, 210
Knowing when to stop, 202, 205
Kuhn's historicist approach, 224–225

Ladder ratings
    assisted living, 40, 41, 50–51, 51–52
Landers, Ann, 116
Late-life demographic trends, 112
Life expectancy, 70, 105
    at age 65
        healthy and unhealthy, 76
    at birth
        healthy and unhealthy, 75
Life threatening health problems, *see
    also* Health conditions
    coping, 133–134
Life with and without disease, 77–78
Likert-type indices
    assisted living, 34–35, 41, 51–52
Listening to the body, 205
Little things
    assisted living, 48–49, 51
Living with it, 198–200
Longitudinal patterns of change
    factors affecting, 95–100

MacArthur Studies, 111
MacArthur Studies of Successful Aging,
    2, 83–103
Managing everyday life model, 181–208
    analytic techniques, 189–190
    implications, 204–208
Managing pain
    strategies, 167
Masoro, Edward, 1–2

Masoro Review
    of successful aging, 59–61
McLuhan, Marshall, 220
Measures
    used for successful aging study, 6–
        11
Medication routines, 192
Medium is the message, 220–227
Mental health, 7
Metanarrative analysis, 220
Metanarratives surrounding successful
    aging, 220–227
Military populations, 108
Modifying effect
    comorbidity, 169–170
Monitoring, 200–202
Morgan, David, 187
Multiple chronic conditions
    role do patterns, 210–212
Multiple chronic health conditions
    coping with, 209–219
    managing, 181–208
Multiple health conditions, 118
Multiple regression analyses, 43–44
Multiplicative effect
    comorbidity, 169

National Health Interview Survey
    (NHIS)
    age-specific estimates, 72
    data, 107–108
Neighborhood and financial problems, 10
Neomodernism, 224–225
NHIS
    age-specific estimates, 72
    data, 107–108
Nonlife-threatening diseases, 130–134
Nonlife-threatening health problems
    coping, 133–134

Obesity, 22
Old age activities, 15–16
Optimization, 114
Overdoing, 202

Pain, 130–131, 165
    coping strategies, 166–167
Penrod model, 212–213
Perceptions
    assisted living, 51
Personality
    coping with comorbidity, 127–128
Personal mastery beliefs, 89
Philosophy of science positions, 221–
    224

Physical, 160
  cardiovascular disease influences, 156
Physical decline
  Seeman and Chen's Study, 110–112
Physical dimensions, 28
Physical functioning, 86, 104–115, 110
  levels, 96
Physical health and disability, 6
Physical performance
  multivariate models predicting
    changes, 98–99
Planning ahead, 199
Plasticity of aging, 26
Poon, Leonard
  perception of chronic diseases, 213
  thoughts on comorbidity, 227
Positivism, 221–223
Postmodernism, 223–224
Power of education, 110
Primacy, 172
Primary appraisal, 122
Problem-based coping, 207
Problem-focused coping, 123
Productive aging, 2, 26
Protective factors
  for physical functioning in older
    adults, 83–103
Psychological characteristics, 89–90
Psychological dimension, 28
Psychosocial factors
  functioning, 101

Quality of life, 8–9, 105–107
  comorbidity, 121
  comparisons, 16–17

RA, 84, 165
Race differences
  in length of healthy life, 78–81
Rakowski, William, 65–68
  aging in terms of reciprocity, 227
  thoughts on successful aging, 113–114
Reciprocity
  in assisted living settings, 25–53
  study, 32–53
  definition, 29–31
  importance of, 30
  and successful aging, 48
    bivariate correlations, 42–43
  William Rakowski thoughts on, 227
Reflecting off others, 201
Reflecting on myself, 205
Reflecting on the self, 200

Reinforcement, 171
Religiosity and spirituality, 9–10
Reported prevalence, 107
Resident characteristics
  assisted living, 36–38
Resident interview
  assisted living, 33–34
Responses
  assisted living, 41
Rheumatoid arthritis (RA), 84, 165
Riley, Matilda, 61
  commentary
    successful aging, 61–62
Risk factors, 11, 104–115
  for physical functioning in older
    adults, 83–103
  social-contextual, 124
Roos and Havens' criteria, 2
Routines
  medication, 192
Rowe, John, 1
Rowe–Kahn model, 67

Schmidt's approach
  aging successfully, 3
Schmidt's definition
  successful aging, 113
Science positions
  philosophy of, 221–224
Seeman and Chen's investigation
  change over time, 113
Selection-optimization-compensation
  model, 67
Selective optimization
  concept, 28
Selective optimization with
  compensation, 114
Self-anchored ladder rating scale
  assisted living, 34–35
Self-assessed health, 77
Self-criticism
  stress and coping researchers, 145–146
Self-efficacy beliefs, 89
Self-rated successful aging
  correlates and predictors, 1–23
Senior Olympics
  assisted living, 53
Sex, 11
Slow progression, 195–196
Smoking, 23, 94
Social comparison, 216
Social conflict
  functioning, 101

Social context
  successful coping, 128–130
Social-contextual risk factors, 124
Social dimension, 28
Social networks, 176
  characteristics, 88–89
    assisted living, 53
  convoy, 29
Social prevalence, 121
Social relationships, 9
Social support, 176
  for coping
    cardiovascular disease, 158
  means of coping, 162–164
  role, 29
Sociodemographic characteristics, 87–88
Spirituality, 9–10
Staff
  assisted living, 48–49
  characteristics, 38
  interview, 36
Staying in control, 193–204
  with multiple chronic conditions,
    203–204
Strawbridge, William J., 62–65
  self-rating, 226
  successful aging, 113
Stress
  cognitive-behavioral theory, 122
  and coping models, 212
  and coping researchers
    self-criticism, 145–146
  and coping studies
    strengths and weaknesses, 146–147
  hypothesized coping model, 214
  sources, 193
Stressful events
  chronic diseases, 210
Stroke, 165
Subjective anchors
  assisted living, 52–53
Subjective data, 223
Sublimation, 173
Success at aging
  premises, 27–29
Successful adaptation, 217
Successful aging
  analytic strategies, 11–12
  attributes, 17–19
  Baltes and Baltes' conceptualization,
    114
  concept
    critique, 59–67
    history, 56–58

conceptual definition, 58–59
five-year predictors, 19–21
Masoro Review, 59–61
media's depiction, 2
metanarratives surrounding, 220–227
premises, 27–29
and reciprocity, 48
  bivariate correlations, 42–43
Riley commentary, 61–62
Schmidt's definition, 113
self-rated
  correlates and predictors, 1–23
staff responses, 47–48
Strawbridge and Wallhagen thoughts
  on, 113
studies, 5–23
study
  measures used, 6–11
William Rakowski thoughts on, 113–114
Successful coping
  social context, 128–130
Super elders, 2

Theories
  cognitive-behavioral theory of stress,
    122
  on effects of coping with
    comorbidity, 168–173
Therapeutic interventions, 177
Time course, 130–134
Timescale, 122
Timing, 216
Transfer, 172

Understanding
  barriers, 119–121
Unintended consequences, 55–69
Unknowing silence, 196–197
U.S. Department of Health and Human
    Services (USDHHS)
  quantity, 71–72
Usual aging and successful aging, 26

Vision impairment, 10
Visual impairment, 165–166

Waging a war, 193
Wallhagen, Margaret, 62–65
  thoughts on
    coping reactions, 216
    multiple chronic diseases, 212
    self-rating, 226
    successful aging, 113
Working through it, 198